a
Caregiver's Conversations
with God

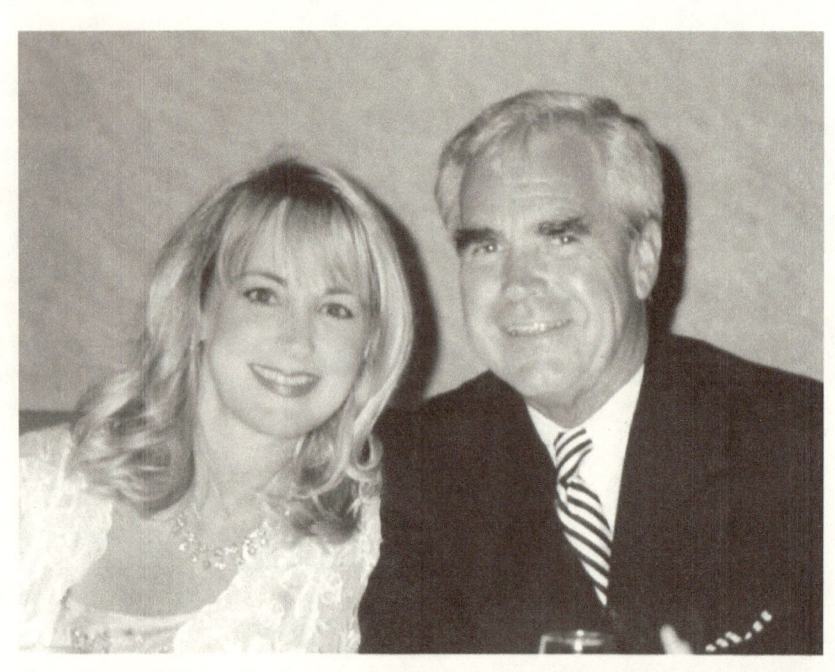

*This book is dedicated
to my heroes and best friends:
My Holy Heavenly Father
and
My Hollywood Handsome Husband*

*Forever and a Day,
Debby*

Copyright © 2018 by Debby Worley
All rights reserved.

No part of this publication may be reproduced or transmitted in any form or by any means, mechanical or electronic, including photocopying and recording, or by any information storage and retrieval system, without permission in writing from the author or publisher (except by a reviewer, who may quote brief passages and/or short, brief video clips in a review.)

For permission requests, write to the publisher, addressed "Attention: Permissions Coordinator," at the address below.

the publishing CIRCLE
admin@ThePublishingCircle.com
or
THE PUBLISHING CIRCLE
Regarding: Debby Worley
19215 SE 34th Street
Suite 106-347
Camas, WA 98607

The publisher is not responsible for the author's website, other mentioned websites, or content of any website that is not owned by the publisher.

FOREVER AND A DAY / DEBBY WORLEY
ISBN 978-1-947398-36-8

Printed in the United States of America

Scripture taken from the *New King James Version*®. Copyright © 1982 by Thomas Nelson. Used by permission. All rights reserved.

Scripture taken from the *New Century Version*®. Copyright © 2005 by Thomas Nelson. Used by permission. All rights reserved.

Scripture taken from *The Holy Bible, New International Version*®, NIV® Copyright © 1973, 1978, 1984, 2011 by Biblica, Inc.®
Used by permission. All rights reserved worldwide.

Scripture taken from *The Holy Bible, New Living Translation*, copyright ©1996, 2004, 2007 by Tyndale House Foundation. Used by permission of Tyndale House Publishers, Inc., Carol Stream, Illinois 60188. All rights reserved.

Book design by Michele Uplinger

A portion of the proceeds received from this book
will be donated toward research
and the cure of neurological diseases.

Contents

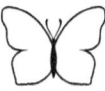

The Beginning 1

First Call. First Date 3

Heaven on Earth 7

Saturday Evening Date 9

Diagnosis Day 13

Communion Comedy 15

Nine and Dine 17

Enough for Today 19

The Love Chapter 21

Matthew 25 23

He Waits for Me 25

Problem Child 27

Backyard Snowflake 31

I Don't Recognize Myself 33

Moving – A Royal Pain 35

Movie Date 39

Flying Your Friendly Skies 41

Special Days 45

The Journey 47

I Need You! Jack Needs Me 49

Sunday Lunch 51

Storms 53

Good News – Bad News 55

Family. Birthdays. Home 59

Jack's Man Cave 63

Still Dancing 65

A Good Day 67

Pharmacy Friend 69

God ??? 71

Just Relaxing 73

Reality? 77

Gift of A Hot Shower 79

Banana Split "Lupper" 81

Cruel 85

I HATE THIS DISEASE 87

Mega Meltdown 91

Alone-Lonely 93

Friends 95

Oh, My Aching Back 99

Struggles 101

Quick Note 103

Basket Dreams 105

Praise Prayer 107

"The Day" 111

Difficult Days 115

Valentine's Celebration 117

Wheels 119

Holding Hands 123

Heavenly Majesty 125

Doors – Thresholds 127

My "Selves" 131

Wedding Anniversary 133

We've Already Spoken 135

Smiles and Laughter 137

Where is My "Want to?" 139

Mountain Worship 141

The Little Magnolia Tree 143

I Love You Roses 145

Jack's Two-Dollar Bill 147

Sweet Sam 149

Missing My Man 153

A Hole in My Heart 157

A Little Weepy 159

Holidays 161

Crazy?! 163

One Regret 165

Sacred, Specific Scriptures 169

Is That Me? 171

The Beginning, Again 173

Author, Debby Worley 177

a Caregiver's Conversations *with* God

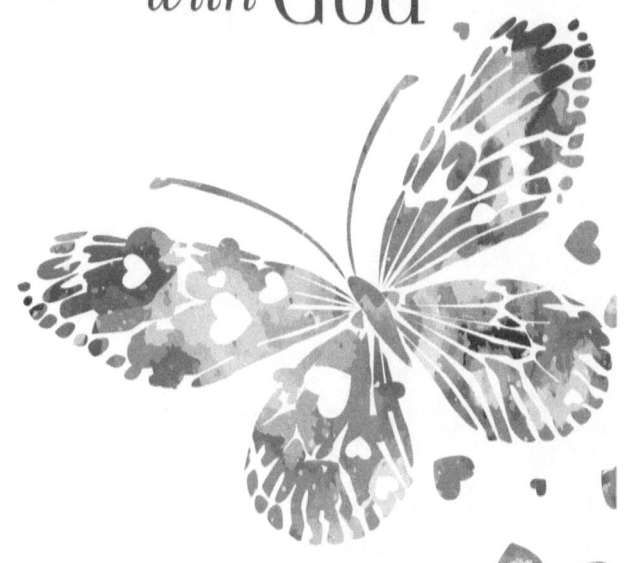

DEBBY WORLEY

The Beginning

Good evening, God!

First Sighting!

    Yesterday was a bright, sunny hot Louisiana day. I was meeting my grown-up children at our local family Italian restaurant—Tony's. I was running a little late. I was wearing my daily "uniform" of faded comfy jeans and a pastel blue top. I walked across the parking lot and noticed a couple of guys walking behind me. Appeared to be a dad-son combo.

    I opened the restaurant door and stepped into a kaleidoscope of familiar decor. Hanging clusters of plastic fruit, yellow and green colored lights dangling from the banisters, red-and-white checked plastic cloths draping the tables. I searched the room for my kids. They had ordered and were sitting in a booth by the window. I smiled when I saw them because they are the best! Beautiful, kind, polite, fun, and crazy like their mom. I handed my purse to my daughter and walked back to the counter to order my lunch. The brightly colored menu is located above the counter. I was concentrating on my choices and decided on two meatballs with marinara sauce and the Greek salad with balsamic dressing. Tony's signature iced tea is a must. Mint leaves are added for garnish, color, taste, and class. Fancy for our small town. In the middle of ordering, I realized the dad-son combo was in line a few feet behind me and technically I had cut in line. I apologized, and the "dad" gentleman said, "You can cut in front of me any time you want!" I joked with them a second, finished my order, and hurried to the safety of my booth.

The "dudely duo" sat close by. The dad sat facing my direction, and I found myself glancing his way, and noticed he was doing the same. We even snuck a smile or two in each other's direction. He was Hollywood Handsome. I was newly single, and men were not at the top of my list. However, something about this Hollywood Handsome man sitting in the booth perpendicular to mine had me "noticing."

My little Louisiana family ate our scrumptious Italian lunch. We laughed, discussed, and caught up on the events of each other's lives. "Dad-son combo" finished before we did and walked past our table as they were leaving. Yep, "dad" was gorgeous up close and personal. Thank You, Jesus, for this little treat for my eyes. The lunch with my family continued with conversation and ended with hugs and kisses. It had been an absolute feast of food, family, and enticing sights. I know, I'm "bad," but sometimes life needs a bit of spice. We all went our individual ways. It was a lovely lunch. I gave myself permission to feel fine regarding the smiles between a complete stranger and myself in the presence of my grown-up children. Besides, I will never see him again.

Thank You, God,
for "best-friend"children, Tony's Italian Cuisine,
and a little eye candy.
Forever and a Day,
Debby

This is the day the Lord has made.
Let us rejoice and be glad in it!
—Psalm 118:24

First Call.
First Date.

Good morning, God!

Remember the "dad" from the "dad-son combo?" He called last night! Two months have passed since our first sighting at Tony's Italian Restaurant. Hence, the person on the other end of the line caught me totally off guard.

He introduced himself as Jack Worley. He said our kids went to school together and shared many of the same friends. I was puzzled until I realized my younger daughter hadn't made it to the family lunch that destined day. So, Jack and I connected the dots. I knew his son's girlfriend, she was my daughter's friend.

After that, we talked for about thirty easy non-stop minutes. He asked me to lunch the next day, noon at Aladdin's. I said I would meet him there, and he laughed. He accused me of having a backup getaway plan. I said, "Yes, a girl can never be too sure, and I always have a backup plan."

After I hung up the phone, I immediately had a mini panic attack. Was it the Hollywood Handsome "dad," or someone totally different? Oh, my goodness, I had no clue. My mind conjured up other men I had seen roaming the streets, cafés, restaurants, movie theaters, and grocery stores of our small hometown. Yikes! Some were extra scary, deeply creepy, and downright dirty and definitely *not* my type. I talked myself down, and remembered it was lunch and I was meeting him at a local restaurant in my own car! Okay! I'm good? Yes, I am!

My first date in years, and it's truly a blind date. He told me what he would be wearing. A green and beige-striped golf shirt and khaki-colored pants. I started to describe myself and he cut me short: "Oh, I won't have any trouble spotting you." My mind immediately went to "psycho" stalker. Vivid imaginations run in our family.

Throughout our phone conversation, I noticed a pronounced speech impediment—stuttering. I also noticed this challenge in speech didn't deter his charm, confidence, or humor. Yes, I had concluded he wasn't a mass murderer or an escapee from the federal prison. By the end of our talk, I do believe he had me under his smooth southern spell.

Please, God, let it be "dad" man.

We met at noon. The restaurant is small, and the tables are covered in starched white tablecloths with vases of fresh Gerber daisies. I arrived first and was seated at a table for two. A couple of minutes passed, and I heard the door open. I instinctively turned my head a bit before I caught the faux pas of my curiosity. *It was him!* He smiled directly at me, my heart skipped a beat or five, he sauntered to the table in slow motion and the closer he got, the cuter he became. How is that possible? Yep, he's my type.

He asked the waiter to bring iced tea for two and an appetizer of oysters Bienville. We both decided on the avocado-stuffed crab drizzled with béarnaise sauce. We were served in twenty minutes. Our lunch and "get to know each other" conversation lasted two hours. As our lunch wound down, he invited me to the New Year's Eve party at the Country Club which was in two days.

I stopped breathing for a sec. Dating wasn't in my plans. This would constitute a date-date. Dressing up, makeup, hairdo, and uncomfortable mile-high heels. Dancing. Sitting with strangers, including my date! I told him, "Let me think about it and I'll let you know tonight, so you can find someone else if you need to." He smiled and agreed.

We talked last night. I said yes to the suave and debonair gentleman. I'm searching my closet *today* for dress-up clothes and stilettos. *Tomorrow* I'll be dancing the night away with a Hollywood Handsome man at the New Year's Eve bash. He will pick me up for dinner. Reservations at 7 p.m. Band plays from 8–12. I just remembered the part about a kiss at midnight! I may have to practice on the mirror—refresher course. Worked in junior high.

Everything is happening so fast.
Please help me make good decisions.
Please help me have fun.
Please come to the dance with us!
Forever and a Day,
Debby

Shout with joy to the Lord, all the earth;
burst into songs and make music.
—Psalm 98:4

Heaven on Earth

Good morning, God!

My life is heaven on earth and I thank You, God, all day long and I know that's not enough. There are no earthly words to describe how ecstatic I am You sent Jack my way "to have and to hold."

Jack and I have been busy the past couple of months. You shared in all our joys!

Romantic engagement dinner and dancing at home, just the two of us. The gift of his mother's ring.

Our wedding ceremony was a month later, March 5, at The Sunset, an ancient, romantic red-brick building downtown. Ancient and romantic just like us! Our kids were concerned about our promptness, but we are "old farts," and know a thing or two about love. We did instruct them to never ever under any circumstances do what we had just done. Marry your soul mate after just three months of dating!

I wore an elegant, long *white* wedding gown with a beautiful veil adorned in pearls. I don't follow the rules that often. Well, I do try to follow Yours as closely as possible. Anyway, Jack wore a black tux with a classic white shirt, and beautiful gold and black onyx cuff links I had given him as a wedding gift. We looked gorgeous! I was the fairy-tale princess walking down the rose-petal strewn aisle toward her hunk—Prince Charming.

Family surrounded us and shared in the beginning of our new life together. After the "kissing," our families joined hands and formed a circle. Each one lit a candle and placed it on the simple, yet elegantly decorated table, that represented a bond of oneness as a blended family. A prayer was offered. Feasting and dancing began immediately!

Our first dance was Rod Stewart's, *Have I Told You Lately That I Love You*. Such a perfect song with perfect words for perfect partners. Can I get anymore sappy? Yes, I most certainly can. We decided to tote the wedding party about two miles away to GG's. Our dance home away from home. The one in the questionable part of town Jack introduced to me on our first date-date. We arrived decked out in our wedding attire, and questionable was highlighted!

Fun! So much fun!

The band pulled us on stage and danced with us. Wonderful to see our family dancing like no one was watching. Not to say our family members can't dance. But there are a couple, and You know who they are. We danced and loved the night away.

My life is heaven on earth and I thank You, God, all day long and I know that's not enough.

Forever and a Day—
we will love each other,
we will love You,
Jack and Debby Worley

You changed my sorrow into dancing.
You took away my clothes of sadness,
and clothed me in happiness.
I will sing to you and not be silent.
Lord, my God, I will praise you forever.

—Psalm 30:11–12

Saturday Evening Date

Good morning, God!

Thank You for love! The human kind of love between a man and a woman.

The kind of love I've found with the man of my dreams.

I love him. He loves me. Passionately and perfectly in our own imperfect way.

Last night is a heavenly example of "Jack and Debby" love. We dressed up for our Saturday Evening Dinner Date. Every Saturday. Seven o'clock reservations at Mazen's Mediterranean Restaurant.

Jack wore his black hound's-tooth tweed jacket, knit shirt, and black pants. His favorite Cole Haan loafers with cool patterned socks. Dashing.

I wore my long black velvet dress. Long dangling crystal earrings and matching bracelets. High heels, of course.

We left the house at 6:45, arriving on time. Samantha escorted us to "our" table. Little gem for two tucked against the wall. Fresh wildflowers in a petite vase, and a lit candle adorned the white cloth. Jack escorted me to my seat. He ordered our Pouilly-Fuissé and crab crepe appetizers. While the waiter busied himself with our order, Jack reached for my hands. We smiled at each other, and quietly talked about our day, our dreams, our kids, our future. We laughed and teased. Life with Jack is easy and effortless.

Our drinks and appetizers arrived, and we continued our Saturday romantic dinner.

Entrees followed. Toasted trout almandine, topped with lump crabmeat and lemon-butter sauce, sautéed spinach, and kibbeh dipped in hummus. We lingered over every course. No need to rush. Tasting each bite is pure joy!

Most patrons order Grand Marnier soufflés for an elegant dessert or bananas Foster prepared tableside. Most patrons drool just anticipating the first bite. Not Jack. After a leisurely romantic dinner, and an exquisitely prepared feast of exotic cuisine, Jack pays the waiter, stands, pulls my chair out, and takes my hand. We wave to friends we see dining on their perfectly prepared soufflés.

We walk to the car. Jack opens my door with his Southern Gentleman Style and I slide in.

Jack gets behind the wheel and does a donut at approximately fifty miles an hour while he puts the car in reverse. Tread marks are left. I know the plan and the routine, so I'm not surprised. I love this part of the date. We speed down the highway, back roads, and shortcuts and swing into the first open stall of Sonic. Jack rolls down the window and is usually hyperventilating at this point. He presses the red button on the menu board and proceeds to order our exquisite dessert for the evening. He's usually a tad amped up by this time, so the stuttering surfaces a bit, but Jack handles it beautifully. Two hot fudge sundaes with cherries on top! Two minutes pass and a skating waitress in short-shorts delivers our desserts served in clear plastic cups. We sit back in the comfort of our bucket seats and savor each bite with our white plastic Sonic spoons.

That's one of my favorite features of Jack. He enjoys life. He doesn't try to impress. Arrogance isn't in his vocabulary. Fun most definitely is! Life is a continual surprise. I'm already looking forward to next Saturday. Our little love ritual. Life is wonderfully delicious.

Thank You for my unpredictably-predictable fun husband!
Forever and a Day,
Debby

*Love puts the fun in together,
the sad in apart, and the joy in a heart.*
—Anonymous

Where there is love there is life.
—Mahatma Gandhi

*Once in a while, in the middle of an ordinary life,
love gives us a fairy tale.*
—Author Unknown

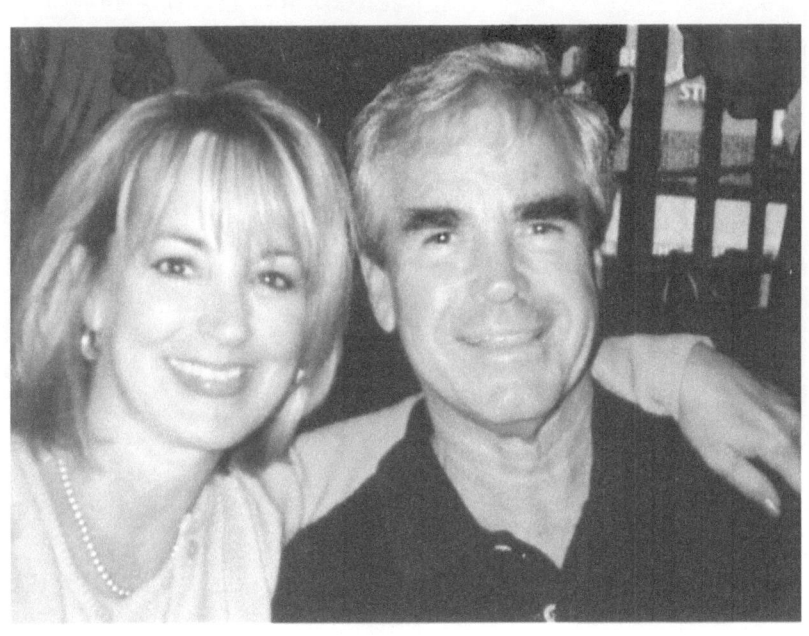

Diagnosis Day

Good morning, God!

Thank You for walking with us this past weekend. Beginning early Friday.

Diagnosis Day.

After months of doctor visits, to determine the reason for Jack's symptoms and many months of REM sleep tests, night terrors, bloodwork, and hand tremors, we were given an answer.

A neurologist tested, retested, probed, questioned, listened.

Then, he called us into his office.

In a professional, matter-of-fact manner, he delivered and explained the news.

"Jack has Parkinson's."

How? Jack was the picture of perfection. Handsome, fit, intelligent, and clever.

Diagnosis confirmed.

Parkinson's and Lewy Body Dementia.

We were silent on the drive home.

We thought about the news for a second. Then we did what most "normal couples" would do under the circumstances.

We packed our bags, climbed in the car, cranked up the music— *Ride Sally Ride*.

We *Hit the Road Jack*. No looking back. Not now. Not yet. We ran away.

New Orleans. Our home away from home. Our destination. We escaped the news, the mandate, the sentence handed down to us by a movement disorder doctor about two strange, new (to us), unwanted illnesses.

We decided to "pass a good time" for three days and two nights. The Windsor Court. The Big Easy. The city we both loved. Hand in hand, we walked the streets of the French Quarter and Jackson Square. Said a prayer at St. Louis Cathedral. We jumped on the St. Charles streetcar and rode Uptown.

Breakfasts were spent outside, eating powdered beignets and drinking coffee with chicory under the green-and-white striped awning of Café Du Monde.

During the day we climbed in a horse-drawn carriage and took in the beauty and intrigue of this fascinating city. We visited our favorite restaurants: Galatoire's, Antoine's, Commander's Palace.

The evenings were romantic and endless as if we were running from something and toward each other. Music filled the air and we danced in the streets to *New Orleans Lady*.

We held each other, we laughed continuously, we cried a little and we promised again to stand by one another "in sickness and in health."

Thank you, New Orleans. Thank You, God.
Forever and a Day our love.
Debby and Jack

PROMISES

... To have and to hold
from this day forward,
for better or worse,
for richer or poorer,
in sickness and in health,
to love and to cherish
all the days of our lives ...

Communion Comedy

Good morning, God!

It's Monday morning, and I'm *still* smiling out loud about something Jack said yesterday at church in the ultra-reverent sanctuary. I imagine You still have a smile on your face as well.

Just to reminisce . . . We were sitting obediently on the long wooden bench, second row from the front. Meditating, singing, listening, we were perfect little members. Communion was next on the program. When it was our turn to walk single-file down the middle aisle, we took our place. Heads bowed, hands folded. We approached the priest. He held an intricately etched chalice filled with wine, and an ornately decorated silver tray layered with unleavened bread. The soft organ music played in the background. A beautiful setting. A quiet (as a church mouse) moment.

After dipping our wafer in the wine and "partaking", we filed back to our spot on our row. I sat down in my designated seat, and Jack sat next to me. As he sat, he looked down at his brand new cream-colored starched linen pants where there was a noticeable red wine-colored spot the size of a silver dollar. I turned my head toward him at the exact moment *the word* came out of his mouth. "Shit!" It did not register as a whisper, more like a trumpet from the choir loft. Our eyes were fixed on each other as we froze for a second. Without missing a beat, Jack tried to recover: "Holy shit?" We just stared at each other, held our breath, tried to process the predicament, and then these perfect little church members began to laugh. Muffled laughter that began with shaking shoulders (no Parkinson's necessary) and evolved into silent laughter that produced tiny drops of sweat even in a cold cathedral.

I don't need to remind You we were so close to the priest he could have touched us (or slapped us). Thank You the service was almost over, and the priest just needed to pray and bless us—if we were still on the list.

After the service, as we were walking to the car, Jack asked, "Do you think God is mad at me?" I said, "No, I think you made His day."

The moral of our memorable adventure? A little hand tremor can bring on an event that will provide smiles and laughter from here to heaven. Our response? You're welcome!

Thank You for loving us and forgiving us when we accidentally cuss and laugh in church on the same day! You're the best.

We love you,
Forever and a Day,
Jack and Debby

When all the wine was gone, Jesus' mother said to him, "They have no more wine." So, in Cana of Galilee Jesus did his first miracle. There he showed his glory, and his followers believed in him.
—JOHN 2:3, 11

Yes, all have sinned; all fall short of God's glorious ideal; yet now God declares us "not guilty" of offending him if we trust in Jesus Christ, who in his kindness freely takes away our sins.
—ROMANS 3:23–24

Nine and Dine

Good morning, God!

Gorgeous golfing weather is in the forecast for the day! It's Thursday and Couples Golf Night at the Club. Four o'clock sharp. The evening and event is titled "Nine and Dine." We play nine holes and then meet inside for Cajun cuisine. Awards are presented during dessert with a beverage of your choice. My choice is chardonnay, Jack's choice is always Sprite.

People can be insanely serious about golf. Jack and I have been on a winning streak. Our title must be defended tonight! Yes, we can be insanely serious on occasion.

Jack will take a power nap, from one to three. I am his alarm clock. He will take his meds and we'll drive four blocks, arriving at the Golf Club exactly as scheduled at 3:30. Our golf cart and clubs are ready for us—yes, we are spoiled. We warm up for a few minutes. We head to the putting green and top off our practice by discussing strategy. Tremors and rigidity must be factored into the equation. Carbidopa-Levodopa kicks in right about this point in the game plan. Timing is everything!

Jack is a quiet kind of fierce competitor. He's tried to teach me golf etiquette. I've improved. My screaming is softer, and I cover my mouth when I yell, and I jump up and down much less frequently. I wear cute outfits, so that should count for something.

Jack has the long game down, and I take over with the short game. Especially chipping and putting. Jack's tremors cease the instant he grips the golf club, and he hits the ball with the ease, distance, and accuracy of a pro. He hits it so far, we usually just need an eight iron to reach the green. That's when I take over with my magic! Jack taught me the short game, and I'm an excellent student. Jack brags about my knack for the game to anyone who will listen. I do love the game, the places we visit, and golfers who have become best friends. Golf has introduced me to a new world of interesting people, magnificent scenery, exotic destinations, and unforgettable memories with Jack.

I love being outside with friends, Jack, You, and Your creation. We meet interesting critters on our Louisiana course. Alligators, foxes, rabbits, egrets, red-headed woodpeckers, and giant mosquitos sunning on the greens and by the bayous. Azaleas are in bloom and so breathtakingly beautiful.

Golfers gather at four o'clock for instructions and format information. Let the games begin!

With a few adjustments, we are learning to live with this mysterious disease and win a few first-place trophies with bragging rights. Our friends don't know about Jack's illness. He has sworn me to secrecy. So, the win is always that much sweeter! When the winners are announced, we kiss, accept our prize, and share a special wink.

> Thank You for gorgeous golf weather.
> Thank You for Your stunning creation.
> Thank You for living and winning.
> Forever and a Day,
> Jack and Debby

Sing a new song to Him; Play well and joyfully.
—Psalm 33:3

Enough for Today

Good morning, God!

We had a major discussion this morning. You opened my eyes to truth. Your wisdom has penetrated my soul. Your presence, Your voice, Your reassurance, and Your gentleness—I witnessed these treasures this morning as I stood in the middle of my prayer room pouring out my concerns to You.

Arguing, crying, discussing, bargaining, and pleading, with You—the God of All Creation. Jack has always told me, "I've never heard anyone talk to God like you do." I have no clue if he considers it a compliment or criticism. I'm scared to ask him so, I haven't, and I won't. Well, it's a good thing he was still asleep upstairs, because he would have been blown away by our ongoing bantering. I know I was.

The topic of conversation was money—well, lack of it. Finances . . . medical bills stacked on the desk, household bills filed in folders, hospital payments glaring me in the face, stock market choices plummeting, and savings depleting as we speak.

A miracle happened in our designated prayer room this morning. As I was pleading my case, and presenting our dire situation crying so violently, I can't believe I was able to hear "Your Voice." A gentle whisper asking me, "Do you have enough for today?" I stopped for a brief second and turned my head toward the direction of the whisper. Then, I continued to argue and cry and add additional valid reasons to be petrified I didn't have the finances I needed to take care of the man I loved. Once again, You calmly and patiently said, "Do you have enough for today?"

At that moment, I knelt on the floor and asked for forgiveness. My response? "Yes, Lord, I have more than enough. Please forgive me." Replacing my frantic "what ifs", I entered a peace beyond all understanding, one of Your top ten promises.

You continued to speak to me. You reminded me of the heavenly manna You sent daily to Your children in the desert traveling to the Promised Land. You supplied their daily needs.

You brought to remembrance my favorite "magic" Bible story as a child. The woman and her son and Elijah. There was a famine in the land. Elijah was a stranger, yet she shared her last meal with him, and You know the rest of the story. Her jar of flour and the jug of oil never ran out until the famine was over. You supplied her needs, one day at a time, day after day after day. Even the Lord's Prayer mentions "give us this day our *daily* bread."

Thank You for spending this incredibly amazing spiritual experience with me this morning. I will *never* forget. Thank You for listening, answering, and opening my eyes to Your truth and promises.

Thank You! We have *more* than enough for today!
Forever and a Day,
Debby

The jar of flour and the jug of oil were never empty just as the Lord, through Elijah, had promised.
—1 KINGS 17:16

My God shall supply all your needs according to His riches in glory by Christ Jesus.
—PHILIPPIANS 4:19

The Love Chapter

Good afternoon, God!

> *If I speak with the tongues of men and of angels,*
> *but have not love,*
> *I am only a resounding gong or a clanging cymbal.*
> —1 CORINTHIANS 13:1

You've opened my eyes once again through the scriptures. That still, small voice reminded me of a specific verse that applied to me . . . and not in an attractive way, I might add. Thank You very much! Nonetheless, it was exactly what I needed. Then, like You do so often in my life, You repeated the verse through another avenue a day or so later. To reinforce, remind, and reiterate the verse was indeed intended for me. First, You delivered this verse privately, and then again yesterday at a friend's funeral. Right on our time-frame of confirmation. Even the pastor said he would be reading from a passage not often used at funerals—1 Corinthians 13:1—The Love Chapter!

So, I knew You were telling me to listen and take note that it was in many ways the answer to prayers, sadness, and frustration. The beginning. The answer. The way back in my personal relationship with my husband.

Jack's neurological disease, personality shifts, disturbing comments, and financial decisions reflect his ever-progressing illness. I know this, but many times I feel so hurt, angry, and resentful. Times are extremely difficult. Jack changes from one minute to the next, and I react negatively or not at all.

I pull back. I say things I wish I could toss to the bottom of the ocean.

I know the "enemy" has used this disease to try to tear us apart. From each other. From You. Lately, he has won a few rounds. No doubt there is a battle in play. I do know I'm tired of the turmoil that takes over—fear, anger, distance, silence—the resounding gong and clanging cymbals. I want to be beautiful, soothing music to Your ears, Jack's ears, and my soul. A heavenly symphony would be a nice improvement.

Thank You for speaking to me, even when the topic You bring up isn't very flattering. I do want the truth. I want to grow every day to be more like Jesus. I want to truly live for You. For Jack. Thank You for the miracles of everyday life, for Your still, small quiet voice that whispers magic and correction. Thank You for loving me enough to open my heart to the truth. Your ways are gentle and giant! Help me now, to examine my thoughts, actions, and words that I will show love to others, especially to Jack.

And now these things remain: faith, hope, and love.
But the greatest is love.
—1 CORINTHIANS 13:13

AMEN!
Forever and a Day,
Debby

Matthew 25

Good afternoon, God!

    I don't have a clear picture of where You want me to go or what You want me to do with my life. I have nothing to give. I want to give You all of me. My path is blocked by disease, illness, limitations. What can I give to my Master, Counselor, Provider, Best Friend, Comforter? My hands are empty.

    I've found myself becoming bitter and resentful. Mad at Jack. Mad at You. Mad at me for being mad at both of you. Blaming Parkinson's and Lewy Body Dementia for taking away my ability to make a difference of any meaning or significance. So, I prayed for an answer.

    I opened my Bible this morning and there "it" was, the answer, so perfect there appeared to be a halo highlighting the holy words. This passage was direct and left no doubts, just facts.

    "I was hungry, and you gave me food. I was thirsty, and you gave me something to drink. I was alone, and away from home, and you invited me into your home. I was without clothes, and you gave me something to wear. *I was sick, and you cared for me.* I was in prison, and you visited me." Matthew 25:35–36

    The people asked You, "When did we do these things for You?" You answered, "When you did it to these my brothers, you were doing it for Me."

    I was sick, and you cared for me! My answer so clearly stated. My purpose defined and outlined. Excitement enveloped me! I can and will serve You. My gift to You is caring for my husband as I would care for You. I do have treasures to lay at Your feet.

My hands are busy. My heart is smiling. You know how I love a plan, and this is heaven sent. As my mom would say, "It's time to get busy."

Scriptures are sacred, specific, and spectacular!
Just like You!
Forever and a Day,
caring for You,
Debby

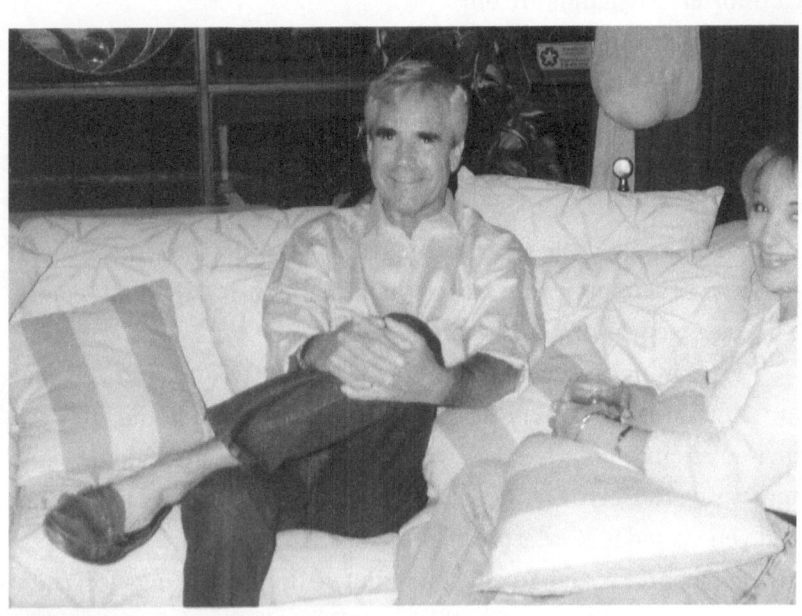

He Waits for Me

Good morning, God!

Snow is falling! Beautiful white doilies from heaven. I'm sipping my Earl Grey tea as I sit in my cozy brown leather chair in a quaint café. Bozeman, Montana. I've traveled hundreds of miles via jet to love and be loved by kids and grandkids. Staring out the window, I remember home and who waits for me: Jack.

Even though I needed this trip, this visit, this "getaway," I find it difficult to relax. I am programmed to care for Jack on a minute-by-minute time frame.

My feelings contradict themselves: peace and worry, happy and sad. You get the picture.

I wonder and worry about small little daily details that can be so monumental for him on his own—tasks we usually accomplish as a "team."

We work together to dress Jack in his accustomed dapper fashion. Clothing choices are purchased with great thought these days, stylish yet simple is our goal.

I sit here and wonder.

How will he open jars, bottles, lids?

How will he be able to climb in bed, scoot down, and put his legs under the covers? How will he pull the covers up to keep his tiny, stiff little body warm? How will he be able to position his pillow without my help?

Will he remember to eat, drink, shower, brush his teeth, shave?

Yes, I know You are with him, and our children will check on him.

I pray he has a fabulous time while I'm away.

My wish for Jack's personal vacation away from his hovering, caregiving wife includes: sleeping until noon, eating when and what he desires, watching ESPN all day and night with a little Kathie Lee and Hoda thrown in, taking as many "power naps" as he chooses, playing golf for hours and hours, and topping off the evening devouring a self-determined number of Blue Bell chocolate bars.

I know I've gone on and on this morning talking to myself and talking to You.

I love our friendship—Yours and mine.

This time of rest is wonderful and necessary. I will soak in joy, love, and hugs during my visit, and when it comes to an end, I will travel home to the one who waits for me.

Time to pack up my journals, prepare myself for the freezing two-block walk. Meeting the kids and grandkids for ice cream! It's minus-eleven degrees and the snowflakes have picked up pace and size. I love my kind of rest! Although I may wimp out and order the hot fudge sundae with extra hot fudge on the side, please!

Forever and a Day,
Love to You from Montana,
Debby

P.S. Would You please remind Jack to take his "magic pill." His clozapine. Thanks.

I will refresh the weary and satisfy the faint.
—Jeremiah 31:25

*But those who wait on the Lord
Shall renew their strength;
They shall mount up with wings like eagles,
They shall run and not be weary,
They shall walk and not faint.*
—Isaiah 40:31

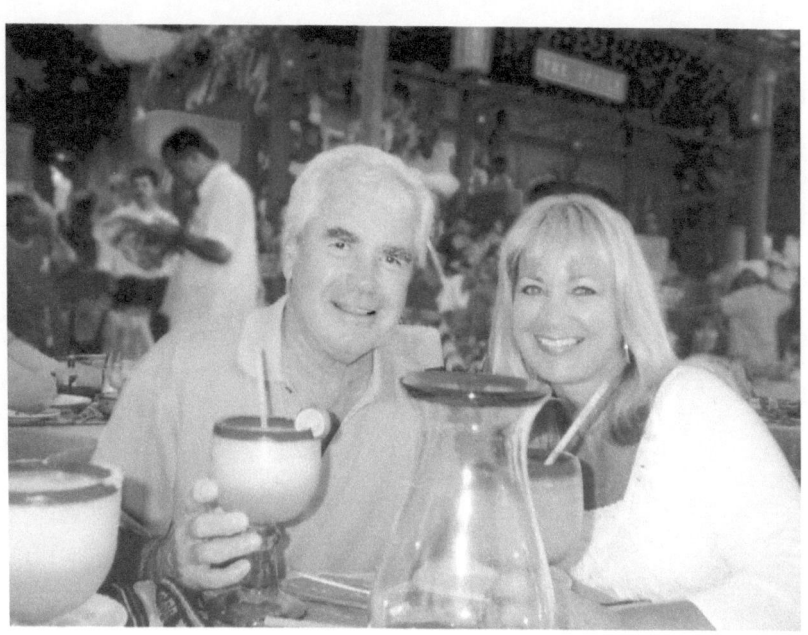

Problem Child

Good morning, God!

It's me—Your problem child!

The last few days I've been overwhelmed, nervous, and scared. So, now I'm overwhelmed, nervous, and scared because I'm overly overwhelmed, nervous, and scared.

Perhaps only You know what I'm talking about.

This is when You say, "Everybody move back, I'm going in to save her again."

Could You step on it? Today is fresh and new and I already need saving.

Go with me. Let me feel words of wisdom, comfort, peace and saving grace.

Okay. I'm feeling much better. I'm ready for this new day. Stay close.

Oops, I'm so sorry. Sorry for being bossy, for giving *You* orders, for not even saying please or thank you! The crazies grabbed me and wouldn't let go. Please forgive me. Thank You for understanding and loving me no matter how overwhelmed, nervous, scared, and *rude* I am.

I love You so much,
Forever and a Day,
Debby—Your problem child

*Do not be anxious about anything, but in everything,
by prayer and petition, with thanksgiving,
present your requests to God.
And the peace of God, which transcends all understanding,
will guard your hearts and
your minds in Christ Jesus.*
—Philippians 4:6–7

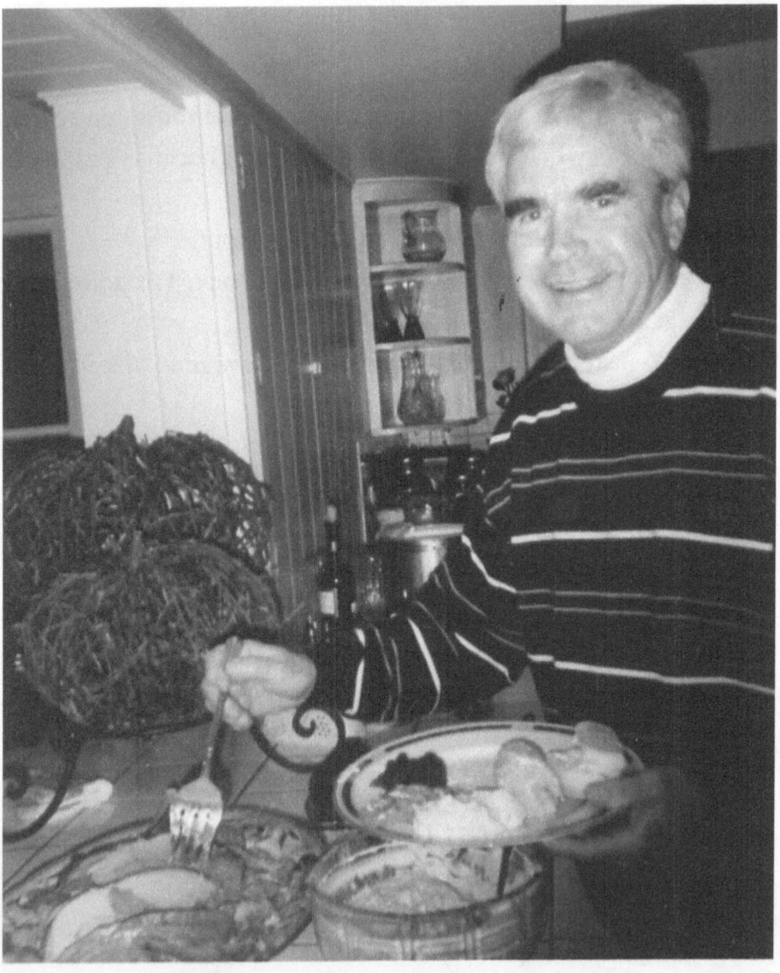

Backyard Snowflake

Good morning, God!

I was out in the backyard marveling at Your creation. The sun was waking and there was dew on the extra-soft green grass. As I walked around the garden, I noticed something glittering in the branches of the pear tree. As I looked up, I saw a perfectly shaped spider web—a sparkling summer snowflake.

Nestled in the silky web was a tiny, fascinating creature working as if he had an urgent deadline to meet.

Each segment of the art was an exact stitch woven together to produce a magnificent display of hard work, persistence, and beauty. Thanks for the mental picture that added a sparkle to my morning, with an even brighter message.

My efforts are minuscule. I know that without a doubt. Many times I wonder, "why bother?" I marveled at this itsy-bitsy spider in my pear tree who was up early spinning a complex web one hundred times his size.

May You take my tiny efforts and magnify them to create beauty and encouragement to those You put in my path and under my roof. Jack is still fast asleep. May his dreams be sweet, and his mind be clear. May I be the sweetheart he needs today.

Spotting the spider was a "wow" moment this morning.

Thank You for my garden, my spider, and my pear tree.

Spectacular!

Thank You for my slumbering hubby and a brand-new day. Awesome!

Forever and a Day,
Debby

The Lord's unfailing love and mercy continue,
Fresh as the morning, as sure as the sunrise.
—Lamentations 3:22–23

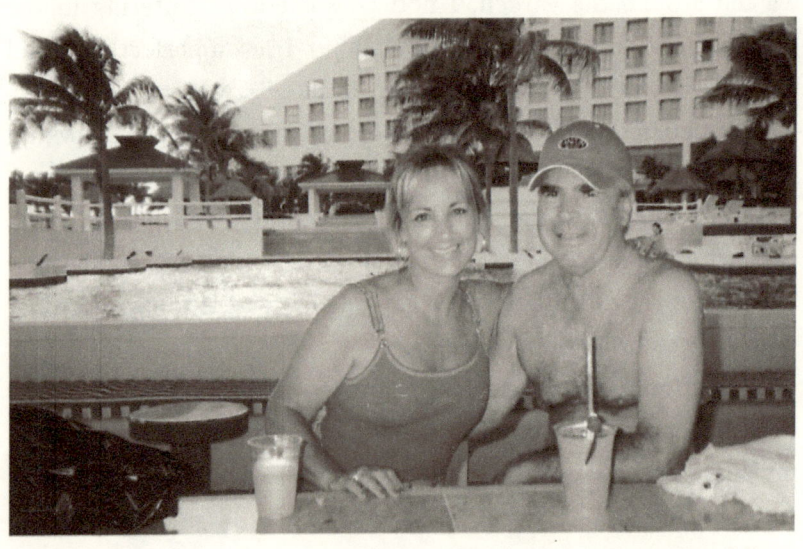

I Don't Recognize Myself

Good evening, God!

Every day is a long day. At the moment, I'm the only creature awake in our little love shack called home.

Another day has come and gone with its good, bad, and everything in between. Sometimes I look in the mirror and I don't recognize myself. And not because I look so hot. My eyes are sunken, dark, and tired. Where is that spark I used to see? Extra makeup is required on a daily basis for this sweetheart. Concealer application makes it possible to move about in public without frightening little dogs and small children. The brush of the thick, beige-colored "goo" does its best to cover the purple, black, and gray indentions under my saggy green eyes. If the eyes are the window to the heart, I need major surgery.

Life was supposed to be easier at this point in my journey. Go figure . . . it's not even close to that prediction.

Tomorrow will be here soon.

I need a fresh pair of eyes to see the possibilities. To feel the love. To reach beyond my situation. To breathe in hope. To lift my hands to heaven. To see the face of Jesus. I know You are close. I just don't feel You at the moment. "Draw near to God and He will draw near to you."

Tonight. Sleep!

Tomorrow. Prayers, miracles, music, family, friends, scriptures,

Jack, and a double dose of concealer!

As *always*, thanks for staying up late, listening, and loving.

I will love You,
Forever and a Day!
Debby

The eyes are the window to your soul.
—WILLIAM SHAKESPEARE

I look up to the hills,
but where does my help come from?
My help comes from the Lord,
who made heaven and earth!
—PSALM 121:1–2

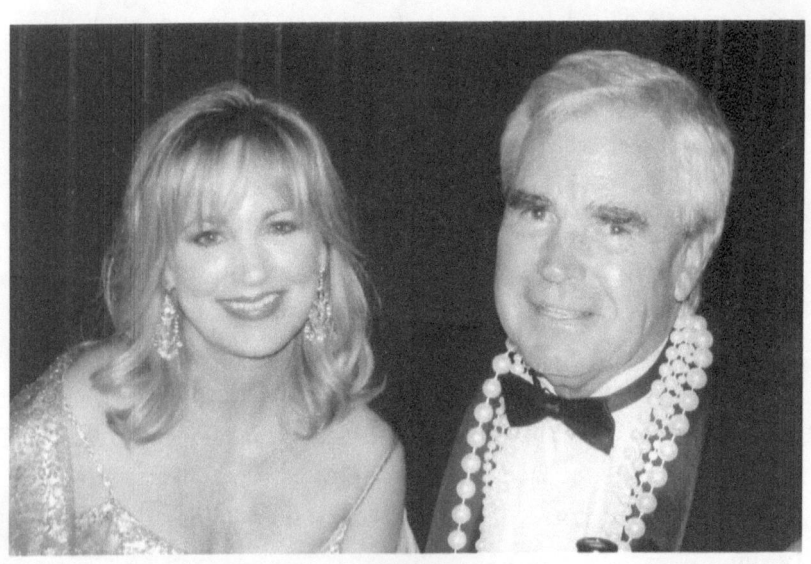

Moving – A Royal Pain

Good morning, God!

I'm sitting in a dark brown, straight-back chair, cozied up at a little wooden table in the corner of the coffee shop. I'm surrounded by a notebook, lease agreement, cell phone, and black sunglasses. My ever-present and expanding "to do list," iPad, and four of my favorite pens are taking a much-needed brake. A large black iced tea, with one teaspoon of sugar, in reach. An oatmeal cookie resting on a napkin, tempting me. I pulled a chair up to the table just for You! Yes, I need You at this meeting, and yes, I'll share my cookie if I must!

I left the house in a hurry, so I threw my hair in a high ponytail. Now my head is throbbing. I knew it would. What's a migraine girl supposed to do on a bad-hair day?

Jack is home watching ESPN. So, I have time for a twenty-to thirty-minute powwow.

Planning a move is strenuous, frustrating, and a royal pain.

As You know, Jack and I will be leaving Louisiana at the end of this month. Jack's home for fifty-plus years, and mine for the last forty-three.

Why do we have to go? Why do we have to move? Why do we have to sift through drawers, closets, pantries, shelves, garages, and memories? Why do we have to say goodbye to children, family, and friends?

We know why. We *still* don't want to.

It all started a couple of months ago with the need to sell our home and relocate. Our bedroom was upstairs, so Jack's unpredictable blood pressure issues pretty much made the decision for us. Fainting, falling, and collapsing down a flight of stairs left no other choice. A professional realtor placed an official "For Sale" sign in our pretty landscaped yard, thus beginning a new chapter in our story.

The housing market was extremely slow. No one was buying. Good for us, because we weren't in a hurry, and we had no place to go. You, on the other hand, had specific plans for us. Always full of surprises! Our house sold at asking price in less than a month!

Meanwhile, Mom was recovering from a massive heart attack in my Texas hometown. She was living by herself, and I wanted to be a part of the healing. I looked into the Parkinson's Community, expert physicians, support groups, medical advances and was impressed with my findings. You knew I would be! I could help Mom, Jack, and find comfort from my family and the exceptional medical field with a single move across the *entire* state of Texas.

I talked to You night and day for a few weeks. Making sure Your hand was in this venture. My mind is clear now and determined to do Your will.

Thank You for meeting me this morning. I've put pen to paper. Pros and cons have been checked and rechecked. You've listened to me, and I've hung on every word You sent my way. I *know* this is the path You need us to take but it *still* tugs at our hearts. It's *still* strenuous, frustrating, and a royal pain.

Time to sign the lease. Time to start packing. Time to call the moving company.

Time for our warm oatmeal cookie and strong Louisiana iced tea! We love You.

We'll forward our new address!

Forever and a Day,
Jack and Debby

*As the heavens are higher than the earth,
so are my ways higher than your ways
and my thoughts than your thoughts.*
—Isaiah 55:9

Not all those who wander are lost.
—J. R. R. Tolkien

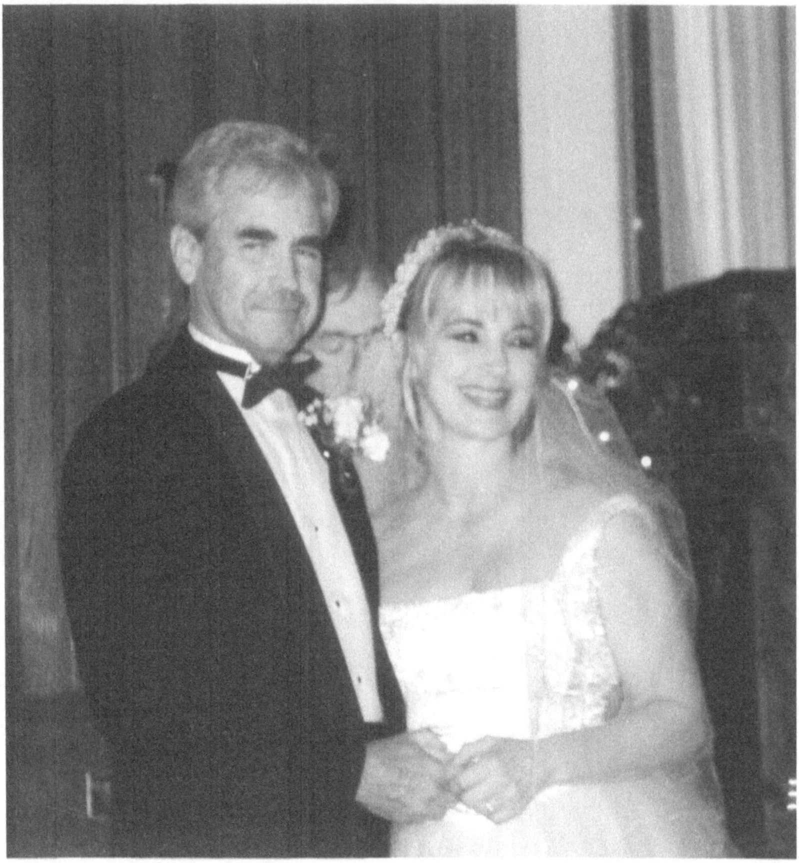

Movie Date

Good morning, God!

Jack and I are in the process of dressing for a movie date. We'll be ready in two to three hours, depending on anything and everything.

Going to the movies to escape for a couple of hours sounds simple, like there should be no problem, but not in our case. Prudent planning is involved. We're becoming experts.

Last week our trip to the theater included unforeseen adventures. We parked in the faded, blue handicapped lane, purchased our tickets, and gingerly found the way to our seats inside theater number seven. I was positive it was our lucky day. When the movie was over, we stood up to leave. We had been sitting for two hours, and Jack's blood pressure became an issue as we walked down the steps of the aisle. We were holding hands and groping in the dark to find our way. I felt Jack's hand and stride become weaker and weaker.

Jack was displaying his "collapsing" position. I possess radar vision when it comes to this specific stance. I noticed the look in his deep brown eyes, the color draining from his thin face, the jerk in his arms, and the hesitation in his step. At that point, there was no doubt: assisted falls were in the near future unless Wonder Wife took immediate action. Then, and only then, would we have a fighting chance to remain upright.

Wonder Wife to the rescue! I braced myself in my super-valiant pose, held him tightly in our standard bear-hug style, and shoved him with all my remarkable powers against the wall— a procedure to brace us from a disastrous tumble.

We held up the line of popcorn-munching patrons as they exited the theater in regular stampede style. No one noticed our predicament, didn't care, or were engrossed in their own daily dramas.

After the crowd dispersed, You did send a nice "stranger angel man" who helped us find a bench so Jack could sit. His blood pressure adjusted. Slowly and cautiously we limped to the car. Short trip. Long walk. Thank You for faded blue handicapped lanes. Silver linings!

Today. Another movie. Another escape. Another day side by side. We're fearless! Grant us secure steps as we venture out into the uncharted territory of early matinees.

We love You,
Forever and a Day,
Jack and Debby

Two are better than one.
If one falls, the other can help him up!
—ECCLESIASTES 4:9

Though they stumble, they will never fall,
for the Lord holds them by the hand.
—PSALM 37:24

Flying Your Friendly Skies

Good afternoon, God!

This morning we were scheduled to catch a flight to see family and friends. Jack woke up and couldn't use his right foot and couldn't walk! "Drop foot!" Another new term. Another new experience.

Somehow, we managed to get dressed, load the car, and drive to the local airport. Another miracle!

As we arrived, panic set in. *Help!* I flagged down a newfound friend. Our dilemma was solved for the moment. Thank you, Stranger Dan, for escorting us to the check-in counter.

One perk we get from using a wheelchair is that we are allowed and (in our case) encouraged to pre-board. Funny how other travelers size you up, some ignore, some scowl, some encourage while others are annoyed and impatient. There were no skycaps available to escort us to our gate, so I decided I was extremely qualified to be the designated "wheelchair chauffeur." Thank goodness for the inconspicuous eight-foot cherry-red pole attached to the side-arm of the wheelchair. We would have gone totally unnoticed otherwise! The entire trip to the gate I remained tangled up with the rotating wheels (only until I remembered to unlock them). Poor Jack was in for the ride of his life and, sad to say, he knew it. My large, stylish vinyl black DKNY travel bag sat elegantly on Jack's lap. You could only see the tip-top of his gorgeous white hair. Looking back, it was probably a blessing for him.

I was pushing Jack with my right hand and dragging our sleek matching carry-on with my left hand. Second thought, there should be training for my chauffeur position. My toes and shins will be scarred for eternity. Jack was jerking from side to side, holding on for dear life at the mercy of my newly acquired skycap skills. We should have split a Dramamine before we began our trek across miles of terminal traffic.

We decided to grab a burger and fries for the flight. We literally crashed into the Pappas Burger to-go entrance and ordered. I (the designated driver) ordered a large adult tea, vodka and lemonade, my new favorite burger drink. Things were looking up. We crashed our way out with *more* to carry. What were we thinking? Don't answer that! I prefer to think of us as adventurous. We were allowed to go to the front of the line because we were sporting a first-class wheelchair. The "gate checker" asked if I had an alcoholic drink in my hand. I replied, "I sure hope so." She didn't appreciate my crazy sense of humor; she didn't even look up. Obviously, she was perturbed and informed me I wasn't allowed to take the drink on the plane. I honestly didn't know this rule. Happily, I am a quick thinker. I put the straw up to my driving hand, puckered up, and sucked that new favorite drink dry. Then this designated chauffeur boarded that jet with my sweet husband and precious pride intact.

As we say in Louisiana . . .

Let the good times roll! (Wheelchair pun intended!)

Aren't You amazed how we find the fun in each adventure?!

Me, too.

Thanks for flying Your friendly skies with us.

We love You,
Forever and a Day,
Jack and Debby

*Be strong and courageous. Do not be afraid;
do not be discouraged, for the Lord your God
will be with you wherever you go!*
—Joshua 1:9

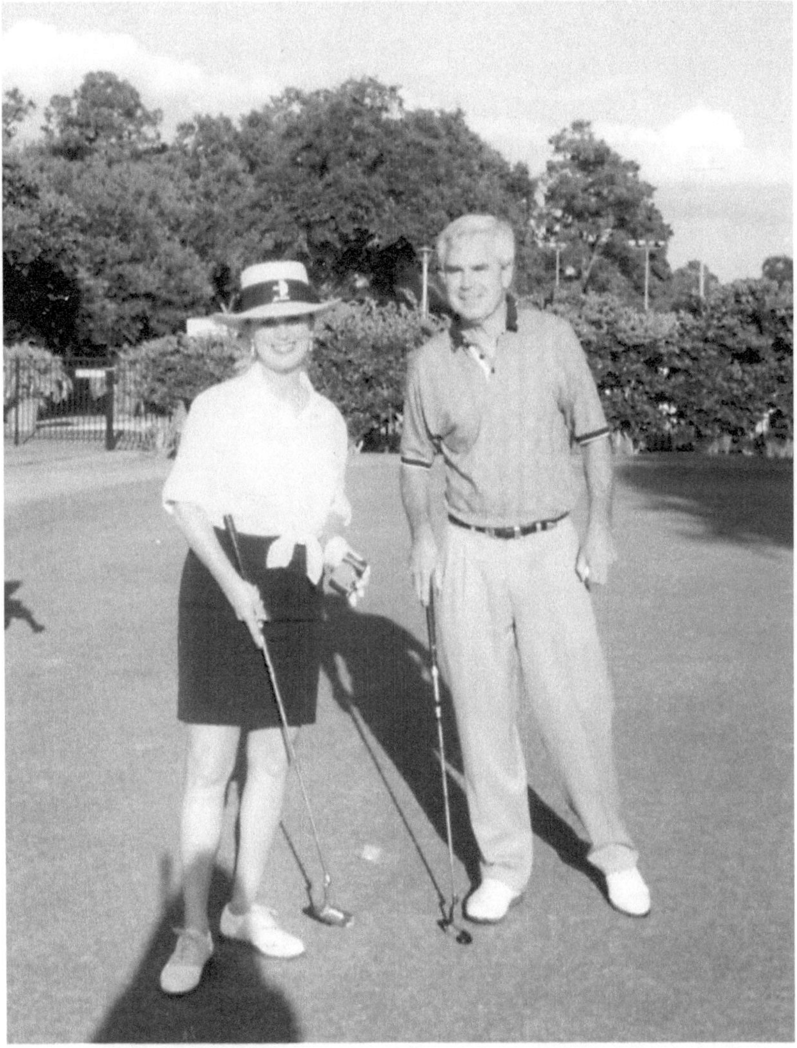

Special Days

Good morning, God!

Today is a special day. Yay!

Today I attend my first Caregivers Support Group. Tomorrow I attend my first Parkinson's Symposium. To most, this would not constitute a stimulating, exciting weekend. Well, they don't know how to spell *fun!* My alarm was set for 7:15 a.m. I didn't need the ringing sounds to wake me. I jumped out of bed at 6:07. Brewed my usual Cajun strong coffee, added two splashes of half-and-half and one teaspoon of sugar. Yum!

My goal is to leave the house by 8:30. Probably won't happen, but at least I have a plan, a goal. Jack may or may not go to the symposium. We shall see when the time comes. Last night, he was totally resistant to this newfound joy of mine. His mind is so intricate, complicated, intelligent, irrational, injured, and fascinating. I never know who, what, where, or when it will present itself and how it might look.

Today is a *special day for me*. I'm going to find my way to a new family. Moms and dads, sisters and brothers, nieces and nephews, aunts and long-lost uncles. Grandparents. I'm stoked! I love them already and we haven't been introduced. I know their heart, but not their names. I'm so excited to meet my new family today, my Caregivers' Support Group.

Right now, I need to prepare Jack's breakfast, a bowl of blueberries, blackberries, and strawberries, with a side of banana-strawberry yogurt, and toast with strawberry jam. Yes, there is a theme here. Strawberries! I'll pour him a glass of orange juice in a small, lightweight cup. The style he can wrap his frail hand around with ease. I'll place these favorite foods in the fridge, and he will eat when he wakes up . . . if he remembers. Morning meds will be lined up on the kitchen counter with a note from his sweet wife, reminding him of the day's activities.

Tomorrow the party continues. Symposium for an entire day! Beginning at nine a.m. There isn't any way on earth Jack will be awake at that hour in the morning. Maybe I can pick him up during our lunch break. Wishful thinking. He'll be watching the Golf Channel if he's awake. That boy can sleep! My feelings aren't hurt. On the contrary. An outing by myself sounds delightful. I am ready to gobble up new information from experts: doctors, nurses, guest speakers . . . all with an abundance of knowledge regarding the newest information, medications, exercise, procedures, and treatments.

This weekend offers companionship, education, and hope.

Sounds magnificent. Let the fun begin.

Forever and a Day,
Debby

"Hope" is the thing with feathers—
That perches in the soul—
And sings the tune without words—
And never stops—at all—
—Emily Dickinson

The Journey

Good morning, God!

This is the continuation of a journey. Much has already transpired, and much is yet to come. I will glance at the past, concentrate on the present, and keep my eyes on the future. Achieving a balance of some sort.

For now there is a calm, but I know with assurance it will not last long.

My days are like roller coaster rides and even roller coasters are unpredictable with the ups, downs, curves, tunnels, darkness, and fear. My eyes closed. My eyes wide open. Gripping the bar, or hands held high. Smiles that can't stop because of the force of the speed. Fear that grasps and won't let go. That feeling in my stomach. My heart pounding and racing and dropping.

I'm holding on like crazy with all my might, and I'm scared to let go. But at times I am so scared I am going to lose my grip out of sheer exhaustion. I've been clasping, holding, and screaming so intensely for oh so long.

You probably don't know what I'm speaking about, unless you've traveled a similar road and ridden a familiar ride.

I never dreamed this ride would take such drastic dips and turns. I pray at times the ride will end. Just end, or at least slow down or even fall off the tracks. But I keep bracing myself for the unexpectedness of the next moment. Knowing without a doubt that it is just ahead. Just around the curve of the tracks.

I remind myself . . . I am strong. I am adventurous. I am lonely. I am scared. I am hopeful. I am confident. I am crazy. I am determined. I am tired. I am beyond tired. I am exhausted. I am a believer. I am a child of God. I am funny. I am a "clean freak." I am very sad. I am desperate.

Just like the roller coaster, I am up and down. I am trusting You, and I am believing in Jesus. I am counting on miracles.

I am finished for now. I will return, for writing is a comfort, a passion, a release, an awakening, and a best friend.

Much love,
Forever and a Day,
Debby

I can do all things through Christ who strengthens me!
—Philippians 4:13

But the Lord stood with me and gave me strength.
—2 Timothy 4:17

I Need You!
Jack Needs Me.

Good afternoon, God!

    I need You! Jack needs me. He counts on me whether he realizes it or not.
    I am his advocate.
    I am his voice.
    I am his warrior.
    I am his love.
    I am his bride.
    I am his encourager.
    I am his interpreter.
    I am his caregiver.
    He is my everything.
    Remember when Parkinson's and Lewy Body Dementia were fresh and new, and I was invincible and strong? My prayer to You was, "Please God, take care of me, and I'll take care of Jack." I would do anything to take back the *years* I tried to keep this agreement with You! Why didn't I let You be God? My strength, joy, sanity, and even will to live were totally depleted. I finally used myself up, and I found myself on the floor crying out for You to please take care of *both* of us.
    You stepped in as I stepped out, and picked me up from the cold hard floor and wrapped me with the strong arms of a Father. You

whispered You had always been with us. I remember apologizing to You and admitting I couldn't take care of Jack or myself.

You gently reminded me I am unprepared to move successfully through life using my own strength. You reminded me I am a fragile human being and You are the one who possesses divine strength.

So, my prayer and my life changed. I can do nothing without Your strength. I know that now. This realization took much too long to soak in and stood in the way of blessings, peace, rest, and laughter. I apologize to You and to Jack. Those days are in the past. Oh, the lessons I'm learning on the path of caregiving.

You are my Wonderful Counselor, You are my Mighty God,
You are my Everlasting Father, You are my Prince of Peace.

I need You. Jack needs You. We *both count* on You.
Forever and a Day,
Debby

The Lord gives me strength and makes me sing;
he has saved me.
He is my God, and I will praise him ...
The Lord is a warrior; the Lord is his name.
—Exodus 15:2–3

The everlasting God is your place of safety,
and his arms will hold you forever.
—Deuteronomy 33:27

Sunday Lunch

Good afternoon, God!

    I have a new favorite restaurant I take myself to after church on Sunday. Someone stays with Jack from 10:30 until 1:30 so I can go to church, grab a bite to eat, and still have time to run to the grocery before heading home to my sweetie pie.
    I usually don't feel lonely or out of place eating lunch by myself but today is different. Everyone is with family, husbands, boyfriends—except me. Insecurity has set in. My waitress is busy and slow at the same time. I order my usual yummy fish tacos, and a to-go burger with fries for Jack.
    She delivers my food in about ten minutes. Perfect! Lunch was scrumptious. I'm usually in and out in about thirty minutes, but not today. My time is precious and fleeting. I need to be on my way, but I can't locate my waitress anywhere. So, I get to watch people talk, laugh, hug . . . and I feel awkward, out of place, and ready to go . . . *where is my waitress . . . where is my ticket?* My brain is yelling at me and reminding me I will be bolting from my table-for-one as soon as possible. I'm trying not to feel sorry for myself, but I need to escape before "sorry" takes me to an entirely new and unattractive level.
    Yay! Here she comes. And there she goes to the family of five! I need relief.
    Okay . . . okay . . . I catch her attention as she is jogging by. Thank you, Jesus. I really mean Thank You, Jesus. I just came from church and I'm still in praise mode.

Finally! She says, "I'll be right back with your check." Hallelujah. Jessica returns with my ticket. Yes, we've been on a first-name basis for the last twenty minutes. I pay her with cash! Big mistake. Ten minutes and counting. Cash always throws things off because no one pays with cash anymore, except me. And I'm paying for it in more ways than one.

Jessica shows up at my table with apologies and change.

I leave a twenty-percent tip as penance for my negative thoughts and a little extra for my busy little server. Who knows what her life is all about? Maybe she needs a break. So, God, please be with my sweet waitress. Bless her. Let her make extravagant tips, and let her customers treat her kindly.

Thank You for helping me through my lonely lunch.

I'm on my way home with a burger and fries for my hubby! Groceries will have to wait 'til tomorrow.

Love You,
Forever and a Day,
Debby

Always be joyful!
Pray continually, and give thanks whatever happens.
That is what God wants for you in Christ Jesus.
—1 Thessalonians 5:16–18

Storms

Good morning, God!

We slept!

Was "iffy" at first. Jack got out of bed a few times in the beginning. I would escort him back. Talking, explaining, praying, hugging, kissing. Placing the mounds of blankets from the tip of his sock-covered toes to the top of his bearded chin. I quietly tiptoed back to my sofa. We were both nice and comfy, then the thunder began shaking the house and bolts of lightning lit up the room. Really? Next the rain and hail did a tap dance on the roof. Really?

I braced myself. Listened for Jack. My fears became reality. Hallucinations were added to the mix of excitement. Storms inside and outside!

He was agitated and started talking to me about the two naked men downstairs. There is no upstairs in our current residence (Mom's itty-bitty home). Then he said, "How could you be swaggering around with two naked men while I'm sleeping upstairs in the same house?" We talked about what he was saying, and I reminded him that with his PD, he could experience situations and people that were dreamlike. He said, "I guess." He had a serious look of disdain. I told him I loved him and spent every minute of the day trying to make his life the best it could possibly be. I would never do anything to hurt him. I showed him the sofa on the other side of the wall where I have been sleeping every night for the last 322 days. He said, "we would see" if what I said was true. He was still upset, disoriented, and angry. I started crying a little. He became more upset with me. I realize he is ill and doesn't have any control over the direction his mind decides to travel. Conversations such as these *still* hurt both of us.

It is 7:30 a.m. Jack is asleep. Hurray! The doctor told me to administer a little extra clozapine last night to see if the dosage would calm the hallucinations. So far, so good. I will be anxious to see if it helps once he is up and "functioning."

Going to make a pot of dark coffee. Enjoy the quiet and hope my caffeine meds kick in before Jack decides to rise and shine.

Thank You, the thunder, lightning, hail, and rain subsided . . . inside. And, thanks, the weather improved outside as well. We survived and slept through the storms once again with Your help!

Thanks for Calming the Storms!
Forever and a Day,
Debby

He stilled the storm to a whisper;
the waves of the sea were hushed.
—Psalm 107:29

I will not abandon you
or leave you as orphans in the storm—
I will come to you.
—John 14:18

Good News – Bad News

Good morning, God!

    Amber, an RN from hospice, came to the house at 10 a.m. to evaluate Jack and determine his eligibility for care with their organization. She is very sweet. I met with her last week.

    Good news and bad news.

    Good news . . . we qualified for hospice care. Bad news . . . we qualified for hospice care!

    We will be assigned Nurse Gloria. She will come by tomorrow and check Jack's vitals, and perhaps draw blood for his clozapine medication. It will be her first visit with Jack. Please let Jack fall in love with her. No jealousy from this sweet wife.

    Chaplain Richard will come by the house Thursday. He will call in the morning to set up a time. I'm ready to pray and be prayed for, Chaplain. Place your hands on us and "do your thing." We welcome you with open arms.

    I pray Jack isn't overwhelmed with all the unfamiliar faces and appointments that will be taking place in the next few days. Once we get into a routine, it will be fine!?! Guess I am trying to reassure myself more so than Jack at this point.

    He is definitely *not* as excited or as cooperative as I am regarding our newfound friends. He still wants to go back to Louisiana and is getting more agitated and aggravated with me as the hours tick by.

    It would be much better if he would talk to me. He keeps his thoughts and feelings inside. His silent gestures, facial expressions, and stubborn cooperation speak volumes. No talking necessary.

I am *tired* and will continue to take extra-special care of Jack. I have finally decided taking care of Jack doesn't mean I have to give up on myself or my health. I tend to forget this daily. I must remind myself moment by moment.

It's time for Jack to rise and shine! This part of the day is delicate. I must tread lightly, cautiously, and tenderly. Any unusual move on my part can instantly end the possibility of a happy morning. So, I tiptoe on eggshells (about six dozen) as I open the bedroom curtains and gently let the sunshine appear through the white wooden blinds. I sit on the side of the bed, place my hand in his, stroke his hair, and "whisper-sing" *Good Morning to You . . . Good Morning to You*. He raises his eyebrows in an effort to pry open his heavy lids. We kiss. I help him out of bed. Our day begins. Success!

Next, my agenda will include serving breakfast. Preparation of breakfast and medications takes place *before* waking Jack. Medications are crushed, poured, and stirred in a shot glass of strawberry preserves. Bathing and dressing are next on our agenda and take about two hours if there aren't any surprises.

Please let there be no surprises. We have an appointment with the neurologist at one o'clock and only four hours to prepare!

Wish me luck and patience and above all *love!*

Thank You for good news.
Thank You for bad news. It's good.
Thank You we qualified for hospice.
Another blessing.
Forever and a Day,
Debby and Jack

*Yesterday is gone. Tomorrow has not yet come.
We have only today. Let us begin.*
—Mother Teresa

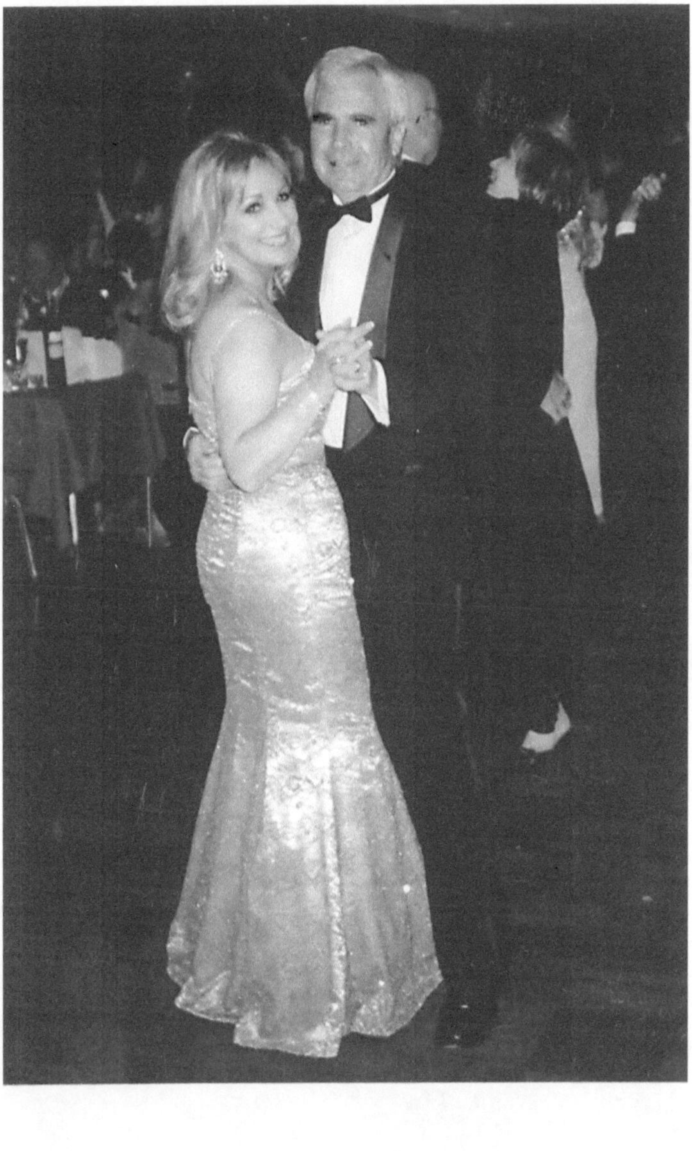

Family. Birthdays. Home.

Good morning, God!

Several updates are tucked in a folder, but I haven't been writing down events nearly as often these days. Not that life has calmed down in the least, I just haven't had the desire or the energy to sit, write, and relive the day's activities. Once is enough! There's no doubt You are my Constant Companion and I speak to You continuously, but writing has taken a backseat for the moment.

Major decisions were made a couple of months ago. Mom continued to improve after her heart attack.

Jack continued to progress in his battle with Lewy Body Dementia.

Jack and I continued seeing specialists, visiting hospitals, and living in rehab facilities.

His disease was relentless and 24/7! I talked to You.

I watched and wept over Jack.

It was time to pack our bags and move back home to Louisiana. So, we did.

Packing, traveling, checking into *another* rehab "hotel" in the hopes of regulating medications, and waiting for "The Cure." August was our check-in date.

Our check-out date is scheduled for November 20. We gave our thirty-day notice. Home for the holidays.

Two days ago, October 22, we celebrated Jack's birthday at his "home" away from home. I picked up ten small Tony's pepperoni and hamburger pizzas with side salads for the shindig. Jack's favorite. Family arrived at five o'clock and Jack sprang to life! Crying and smiling as he hugged, kissed, and held each and every one. We sat outside on the patio and talked, read cards, opened presents, and sang our goofy family birthday song. Jack led the chorus with gusto...

Happy birthday to you,
you live in a zoo.
You look like a monkey,
you smell like one, too.
Oh, yeah!

Entertaining and happy. He was encircled in love.

Family love had chased the blues away for a few moments of pure joy!

Birthday bliss!

Now, back to reality...

It's October 28 at 7:07 a.m. I've been up since 5:30. I tried to go back to sleep, but kept thinking about everything I need to do to successfully bring Jack home. Equipment, people, caregivers, and medications need to be coordinated to make this a smooth transition.

Praying for *divine* inspiration, wisdom, and energy. Poor You, but then again, You knew what You were doing when You put me in this life under these circumstances. I still feel sorry for You. Working with me on a day-by-day basis takes a champion and tag You're it!

Going to finish unpacking and organizing boxes in the guest room today. This is the room I will make Jack's "man cave." Busy day ahead.

Thank You for celebrations,
Thank You for family,
Thank You for home... wherever that may be.
Forever and a Day,
Debby

Life takes us to unexpected places . . . love brings us home.
—Author Unknown

Every day is a journey, and the journey itself is home.
—Matsuo Basho

Jack's Man Cave

Good morning, God!

    Jack is coming home in a couple of weeks. At the end of the month. He's been staying in a "hotel room" until the doctors tweak his medications. I stay every day with him, and sleep at home every night. I'm extra excited he's coming home. However, there is work to be done.

    I have errands to run, phone calls to make, and items to purchase. Medications to buy, caregivers to interview, hospice to co-ordinate.

    My mission is to turn the guest room into an incredible "man cave." A place my husband will call home. A place he feels safe. A room without "monsters." A place only "happy hallucinations" are allowed. A bedroom filled with Your presence.

    Usually, I love to decorate our house. This project is more of a challenge, and at the same time a pleasure. The guest room needs to be totally transformed. The carved wooden queen-size bed must be replaced with a basic twin-size hospital model. Furniture must be arranged and rearranged to create a safe haven. After I work my magic, Jack will come home to a swanky luxurious suite with just the right touches to let him soak in love from every corner and every nook and cranny.

    The challenging part is adding the right mix of memorabilia. So many pictures, artwork, and wall hangings can cause panic and paranoia in a heartbeat. So, it will be trial and error until we arrive at the perfect combination for the perfect "man cave," the perfect "love nest."

I've settled on a chocolate brown and golf-green color scheme. There is a picture of Jack, at the age of five, nestled with his pretty-as-a-picture mom, displayed on the wall at the foot of his bed. A painting of the eighteenth green from his favorite golf club hangs within view. A few books: Bobby Jones, Tiger Woods, Ben Hogan, and his Bible are stacked on a side table. Above his desk hang two framed score cards . . . two of his three hole-in-ones. A family album stuffed with old and new photos is nestled in his drawer. A familiar golden cross sits on his dresser and faces his direction to remind Jack of You.

Yesterday I purchased a high-back wicker chair that fits perfectly between his bed and dresser. A little space for me to sit, visit, hold hands, and steal a kiss every now and then.

Okay. It's finished. It's complete. It's beautiful. Thank You for guiding me and my mind and my decisions as we prepared a perfect place for our awesome Jack.

Please be in our home, in Jack's new bungalow, in his marvelous "man cave."

I love You, Lord.
Forever and a Day,
Debby

I will not go home to my house, or lie down on my bed,
or close my eyes, or let myself sleep
until I find a place for the Lord . . . and Jack.
—Psalm 132:3–5

I go to bed and sleep in peace,
because Lord, only you keep me safe.
—Psalm 4:8

Still Dancing

Good morning, God!

    Thank You for rest. My mind can relax and remember.

    Weekends remind me of happy sweet memories with Jack. Our weekend routine . . . my, how that has changed.

    The dancing. I loved our Friday night dinner and dancing dates. After dinner, we'd find our way to the dance hall downtown and "cut a rug." The band was live and so were we. We danced until the last song of the night was played, even when Jack's legs and coordination were not cooperating.

    Jitterbug. Our favorite.

    Jack was such an incredible dancer. He was so smooth. I just listened to the music and followed his lead, knowing he always made me look as if I knew what I was doing. Jitterbug wasn't my generation's dance, but it was our dance.

    He swung me around, pulled me close, dipped me, kissed me, and twirled me all over the dance floor. Sweet, sweet memories. *Those were the days, my friend, we thought they'd never end.* Fast forward ten years.

    We still turn up the music, close our eyes, and remember.

    Now, Jack lies in his reclined geri-chair and I sit next to him in my swivel loveseat, so close our bodies touch. I take his hand. He doesn't have the strength or the reasoning to reach for mine, so I hold his and occasionally he'll tenderly stroke mine with the rhythm of the beat.

The Otis Redding is loud. *Sittin' on the Dock of the Bay* fades out slowly and *Try a Little Tenderness* is next on the playlist. Jack's soul music.

I sing. Jack's eyes are closed, and I watch his legs because I know that every now and then he'll tap his toes or move his feet to the familiar tunes. I smile, but I also feel the sting of tears and squeeze his hand a little tighter. I close my eyes and remember the "good ole days." I can "see" us dancing, holding each other, so in love, having so much fun, and making fabulous memories.

I never dreamed back then that those memories would bring so much comfort ten years down the road.

We're so blessed! We're still dancing! We're still in love!

Thank You.
All our love.
Forever and a Day.
Jack and Debby

To watch us dance is to hear our hearts speak.
—Hopi Indian saying

A Good Day

Good evening, God!

Today was a good day . . . on a Lewy Body Dementia scale. On a scale of one to ten, I'd definitely give it a solid eight. We talked. He remembered my name. He ate well. He was happy. Me too. I started the day serving Jack his usual breakfast-in-bed menu choice. His fruit bowl filled with blackberries, blueberries, strawberries, and banana slices. A slice of oat toast submerged in peach preserves. An LSU cup with ice-cold orange juice. A side of crushed meds mixed with strawberry preserves in a shot glass. Stirred, not shaken!

We teased, watched Kathie Lee and Hoda. He calls them "my girls." Our hospice sweetheart, Kee Kee, came to the house about ten o'clock to bathe and dress Jack. They sang, prayed, and laughed. Jack loves to see her. She is a gift from God to both of us. After Jack was cleaned up and looking quite dashing in a bright red cardigan pullover and black workout pants, Kee Kee pushed him into the living room in his top-of-the-line geri-chair. We said our goodbyes to Kee Kee. She was on the way to her next patient.

Jack reclines in front of the TV and gazes out the living room window. I work around the house, preparing meals, changing beds, washing sheets, vacuuming, and doing anything else that needs attention—especially checking in on Jack!

Jack is "talking" to some of his best friends. He is speaking to Mac, Bubba, and Whitey. Mac is literally in Cabo, Bubba is in Florida, and Whitey is in California. However, Jack "sees" them and talks to them. He picks up the TV remote and "calls" them and has lengthy conversations. He also "plays golf" with them on a regular basis, commenting on the particular hole, putt distance, club selection, notorious number eight, and final scores. His time spent with them is detailed. Often, they play thirty-six holes. Today he yelled at Mac about a good shot. He said, "Bubba, how did you miss that putt?" He belted out a hearty laugh, complaining about Whitey's sand trap shot. Amazing and precise. He *still* plays golf with his best friends from the luxury of his living room.

Matt, his little red-headed, freckle-faced imaginary friend, arrived at five o'clock in the evening. Matt's been "visiting" for about a month now, every evening at the same time. Jack loves the time spent with this little boy. He tells me Matt is ten years old. An actual conversation occurs. Today, Jack was laughing and telling Matt, "You knucklehead, you can't climb on that chair. Get down or you'll hurt yourself."

Supper is served, and Jack's company goes home.

Happy hallucinations and delightful delusions ROCK!! Today was definitely an eight!

Thank You! God!
Sweet dreams,
Debby and Jack

Normal day, let me be aware of the treasure you are.
—Mary Jean Irion

Pharmacy Friend

Good morning, God!

    Yesterday in the pickup line at the pharmacy, I met a precious, tiny lady. She had thick, short, beautifully styled silver hair. She also had dark, perfectly-shaped eyebrows. I noticed the eyebrows, because only You know the uni-brow issues that have plagued my life. Anyway, back to the sweet little lady. And she was little. I'm 5'3" on a good day. The tip-top of her head didn't reach my shoulders. She told me her name was Irene.
    We chatted a minute.
    She was in line to pick up prescriptions for her absent husband, Pete. He stayed back at the farm, and she was in town to run errands. Husbands were our connection. Caregiving was our bond. I fell in love with this precious new friend—instant friendship. Irene told me she needed to visit with the pharmacist about new medications for Pete. So, she let me check out first.
    We said our goodbyes.
    We promised to pray for each other.
    We hugged. Said, "Have a good day" and meant it.
    It seems as if most of my friends these days are strangers. Strangers who become friends. Thank You for sending these amazing people into my life and for the bond and beauty of pharmacy-line friendships.
    Thank You for opening my eyes to the strangers and miracles

You place right in front of me each and every day.
Please bless Irene and her husband, Pete, back at the farm.

Forever and a Day,
Debby

The only way to have a friend is to be one.
—RALPH WALDO EMERSON

*Keep on loving each other as brothers and sisters.
Don't forget to show hospitality to strangers,
for some who have done this have entertained angels
without realizing it!*
—HEBREWS 13:1–2

I do desire we may be better strangers.
—WILLIAM SHAKESPEARE

God ???

FORGOTTEN!!!!!!!!!!!!!!
Please send help.

We love You,
Forever and a Day,
Debby and Jack

*Troubles have come again and again,
sounding like waterfalls.
Your waves are crashing all around me.
The Lord shows his true love every day.
At night I have a song,
and I pray to my living God.
I say to God, my Rock,
"Why have you forgotten me?
Why am I sad and troubled . . . ?"*
—Psalm 42:7–9

*Why am I so sad?
Why am I so upset?
I should put my hope in God
and keep praising him,
my Savior and my God.*
—Psalm 42:12

Just Relaxing

Good afternoon, God!

It's 3:25. I'm sitting with Jack. He's watching a little TV and just relaxing. At least I think he's relaxing.

He's covered in his big fluffy purple and gold LSU blanket, snug as a bug in a rug.

My back is killing me. That's what I get from thinking I'm strong enough to take care of Jack by myself on the weekends. Try to save a little money, and I "pay" for it with a bad back, hip, and leg.

I have tried to find someone to help during the day on week-ends, but most people don't have any desire to work Saturdays, Sundays, or holidays. However, I will find someone as soon as possible. Calling prospective caregivers this afternoon would not be advised, because I don't believe I could form an intelligible sentence.

I'll wait for a fresh new day, and call early.

Jack has been quiet today, but yesterday he hallucinated a lot. The last three nights when we have said our prayers he has recited *Now I Lay Me Down to Sleep*. No hesitating, or searching for words, or stuttering while repeating his childhood prayer.

> *Now I lay me down to sleep.*
> *I pray the Lord my soul to keep.*
> *If I should die before I wake,*
> *I pray the Lord my soul to take.*
> *God bless Mommy, Daddy, and Sissy.*

I've searched for words to describe the first time I heard him recite this prayer. His words were sweet, surprising, angelic, childlike. He usually says the Lord's Prayer. He woke up this morning and told me about a dream he had. Well, with him, it's not a dream. I've come to the conclusion that he does see and talk to real people even when I can't see or hear them. He told me that You took him to see Jesus last night and then brought him home. He also talks about "his" angel. He says, "I don't know her name, but she lets me do anything I want." He has been talking about this for three days. Guess You really impressed him.

My idea of relaxing involves a few steps. Three to be exact. First, I grab my neck warmer and place it in the microwave for one minute and fifty-five seconds . . . a present from my sweet daughter. I wrap it around my neck. It serves two purposes—a hug from my "baby girl," and toasty warmth for my stiff, tense neck. Next, I grab my two ice packs out of the freezer and sit on them. Yes, one for each cheek. At least it numbs my pain for a bit. Lastly, extra-large Menthol Medicated Icy Hot Patches will be placed down my left leg. What is that smell You ask? Just me and my patches. My Chanel No. 5 and menthol mingle for a rare, pungent aroma. Jack is blessed his sense of smell has long since vanished.

Another blessing! My body may be under wraps, but my hands are free. One is designated to hold Jack's hand and the other to hold my full to the tip-top glass of chardonnay.

Yay! We are both comfy. Jack is watching his "new" favorite show, Bonanza. He loves Little Joe. I love Adam. Life is sweet for the moment. So, we'll sit close and enjoy each other's company. Watch a good old-fashioned rerun of a classic western. Jack is humming the theme song! Showtime.

We definitely love You.
Forever and a Day,
Jack and Debby

A CAREGIVER'S CONVERSATIONS WITH GOD

Sometimes the most spiritual thing we can do is rest.
—Adrian Rogers

*Now I lay me down to sleep
I pray the Lord my soul to keep . . .*

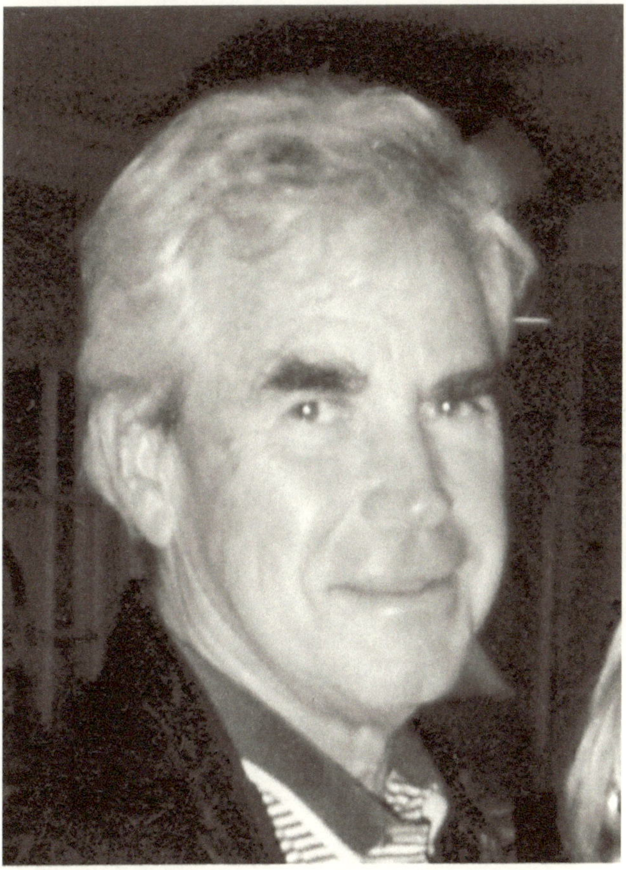

Reality?

Good morning, God!

Hallucinations, fantasies, facts.

I try to explain, rationalize, distract, re-direct, all in the name of *reality*. Jack's dreams, nightmares, hallucinations, and delusions all collide into his scenic panorama called life. It's a runaway train. Traveling faster and faster.

In my effort to help him return from the unknown, I change my mind. I find myself jumping on the first-class passenger car to take my seat next to him. Truthfully, his daily adventures and life experiences are more exciting, dangerous, relaxing, and exhilarating than my life within these four walls called "home sweet home." So, we'll ride these rails together.

I've tried to bring him back from fantasy to reality. Why? He's the one having memorable times: visiting family and friends from heaven, having elaborate lunches with the head of the mafia, playing thirty-six holes of golf every day with Arnold Palmer, Ben Hogan, and Tiger Woods. Water skiing in Lake Tahoe, and fishing for trout in Canada, all in the comfort of his geri-chair in our cozy house.

It's 10:30 and I hear Jack waking. He's calling my name. Although today my name (so far) is "Hey." Yesterday I was "Babe." Perhaps it will be something glamorous by the end of the evening. I also hear the faint whistle of the train in the distance. Where will we go today? Who will we visit? Where will we dine? How many holes of golf will we play?

So, my decision has been made, I'm joining *his* world. I find communication is more enjoyable and entertaining. In *his* world, my days are packed with stimulating events and situations. So, I'm purchasing a lifetime pass and climbing aboard.

He is the conductor the majority of the time. Every now and then, the tracks become bumpy with dangerous turns and rambunctious passengers, and I take charge for a while. I calm the disruptive people on board and find a smoother route. Sometimes we travel several miles down the track before we're in control again.

Overall, our facts, fantasies, and hallucinations have been happy—just the way we like them. At this moment in time, our fantasy *is* our reality.

The train has reached its designated destination for the day.

The last whistle has blown. Passengers have gone their separate ways. We are headed to our cabin for needed rest. The whistle will sound bright and early in the morning.

Reality will begin, again. All aboard!

Thank You for "riding the rails" with us!
We love You,
Forever and a Day,
Jack and Debby

*Man's mind, once stretched by a new idea,
never regains the original dimensions.*
—OLIVER WENDELL HOLMES

*Always have a vivid imagination,
for you never know when you might need it.*
—J. K. ROWLING

And be sure of this: I am with you always . . .
—MATTHEW 28:20

Gift of A Hot Shower

Good evening, God!

Thank You for the gift of a wonderful hot shower.

My heart is heavy, the weight of my pain is excruciating. My shower is a refuge. A place of safety, comfort, cleansing; renewed body, mind, and soul.

Guess that sounds over the top, but remember it's me, and I lean toward the dramatics. However, the gift of hot showers has refreshed me time and time again.

When life seems too difficult to take another step. When I need to cry, but I don't want to upset Jack.

When tears are about to render me helpless and nonfunctional.

When I am surrounded by hospice helpers, and the pain of watching the man I love suffer through heart-wrenching humiliation, fear, and confusion.

Tears begin to well up in my eyes, and I know I must quietly and quickly excuse myself to the extra bedroom. I close the door. Step inside the bathroom. Turn the shower to extra-hot, and climb under the surge of powerful streams of "rain" massaging my body.

Only in that enclosed, secluded space do I allow myself to "let go" and I do.

I cling to the cold beige tiles, I stand under the beating water, and sob, sometimes trying to muffle my cries; other times I have no control over the volume and intensity.

There are times I grow tired of holding myself up, so I sit on the shower floor and allow myself to feel what I feel.

I cry out to You. I only hear myself.

Tears begin to subside. Moans start to fade.

I hear myself reciting scriptures, singing songs of hope, and then feel beginnings of a strange sense of calm. You're here.

Showers are underrated! Many times, I take three showers each day. One in the morning before Jack is awake, one while hospice is helping my hubby with personal care, and one about three a.m. when sleep is evasive, and my mind is "fried."

The beating streams of hot water cleanse and invigorate.

Once again, thank You for the perks, blessings, and luxuries of a wonderful hot shower.

Forever and a Day,
My love for You,
Debby

You have seen me tossing and turning through the night.
You have collected all my tears and preserved them in your bottle!
You have recorded every one in your book.
—Psalm 56:8

The best thing one can do when it's raining is to let it rain.
—Henry Wadsworth Longfellow

Banana Split "Lupper"

Good evening, God!

Early this morning, after my coffee and time with You, I got a head start on the day!

I pulled out the crockpot, roast, potatoes, carrots, onions, olive oil, and garlic. Perfect day to prepare Jack's favorite meal. My favorite, too. Just throw all the ingredients together in one big pot and let it simmer all day! "Lupper" is finished, and it's only 7:45 a.m. Yay. I'm brilliant, happy, and possess a huge sense of accomplishment.

"Lupper" is a word I've made up because our eating schedule has changed drastically over the past couple of years. Once again, we adjust. Adventure is ours.

The word is derived from a combination of two words. Lunch and Supper thus "lupper."

Jack's schedule dictates mealtime. We have found a rhythm of sorts, an adjustable, semi-predictable routine. Breakfast starts about 10:30 and lasts 'til noon (give or take an hour or two). Snack of fruit and mixed nuts whenever his "power nap" is over. Lupper is served from 5:00 to 6:30. Dessert is an essential "side" to his meal.

Today people provided a constant flow in and out of our abode. Leaving the door unlocked works best. I'm not worried uninvited individuals will venture in, because once they see what's taking place inside this residence they won't stay long. So, today hospice friends, Jack's monthly evaluation team, chaplain and chaplain's wife, and the geri-chair replacement equipment gentleman visited.

The roast was smelling heavenly, and I knew Jack would be elated with our menu choice for the evening. Wrong. So wrong.

I prepared his plate, smiling and singing. I placed the lusciously laden dish on his tray and sat next to him. I had a glass of chardonnay in one hand and helped him with his meal with my other. Jack took one look at his plate. Looked at me with disapproval. Turned his head away from me. He was upset. A scowl appeared on his usually stoic face. I tried to coax him into telling me what was upsetting him, and why he wouldn't even taste his favorite meal of all time. Nothing. I picked up the fork and put it up to his mouth, he closed his lips so tightly nothing could get in.

Okay, plan B. I listed everything we had in the kitchen I could prepare for his meal. Still nothing! I was frustrated, tired, and getting nowhere fast.

Okay, plan C. I wracked my brain with possibilities. Then the vision came to me. I could see it vividly. I said, "I know. How about a banana split?" Jack finally turned his head to face me, and a broad smile emerged across his expressionless face! Jackpot! I couldn't help but smile with him. He wears me out, but that look was precious, and excitement was mine as I went with plan C.

Vanilla ice cream, bananas, strawberries, pineapples, chocolate syrup, whipped cream, and a bright red cherry on top. When he saw the large banana split perched on his tray, delight covered his thin, happy face. It's a moment I will always treasure. I brought him a little joy. Oh, by the way, he ate *all* his lupper, so he had dessert! Hot fudge sundae, adorned with whipped cream and two bright red cherries on top.

Thank You for banana split luppers.

Thank You for crockpots, roast, potatoes, and carrots. Thank You I have a head start on tomorrow.

I'm truly ready for sleep.
Long day. Good day.
See You in the morning.
Goodnight.
Forever and a Day,
Debby

*Enter his gates with thanksgiving and his courts with praise;
give thanks to him and praise his name.
For the Lord is good and his love endures forever . . .*
—PSALM 100:4–5

Life is uncertain. Eat dessert first.
—ERNESTINE ULMER

Cruel

Good evening, God!

Cruel!

That's the theme of the last twenty-four to forty-eight hours. I want to run away.

I want to hide.

I want to give up! I want to die!

I wish someone *really* cared.

I wish You would visit, would speak, would take away this cruel time, this cruel disease!

I've been able to move through this illness with Jack for fourteen years now and unless something extraordinary happens, I believe this is as far as I can go.

I can't stop crying, I can't sleep, I can't feel anything but pain and sadness and defeat! I've *really* tried, and I've done my best. The past twenty-four to forty-eight hours have come and gone and I can't do another twenty-four to forty-eight hours like this again. I've had much worse days in the past and moved on into the next day with new hope. I don't see that in the future. Maybe it's around the corner, but it better show itself soon. Hope? Where are you?

I pray deep sleep places its arms around me and heals my soul tonight.

I pray You will take Jack to heaven to live a beautiful, magnificent life, free of this cruel disease.

    Life can be so cruel. Help me hope!

My Love for You,
Forever and a Day,
Debby

P.S. Even on days like today—days I search but can't find You.

I believe in the sun, even when it is not shining.
I believe in love, even when I don't feel it.
I believe in God, even when He is silent.
—AUTHOR UNKNOWN

I find rest in God; only he gives me hope.
He is my rock and my salvation.
He is my defender;
and I will not be defeated!
—PSALM 62:1–2

I HATE THIS DISEASE

Morning, God! No good in it.

> I HATE MYSELF.
> I HATE PARKINSON'S.
> I HATE ATYPICAL PARKINSON'S.
> I HATE LEWY BODY DEMENTIA.
> I HATE NEUROLOGICAL DISEASES.
> I HATE WHAT IT DOES TO A PERSON,
> TO A FRIENDSHIP,
> TO A MARRIAGE,
> TO A SOULMATE,
> TO A RELATIONSHIP,
> I WANT TO SAY I HATE YOU, TOO . . . BUT DEEP DOWN I KNOW I CAN'T BECAUSE YOU ARE MY ONLY HOPE. SO, I GUESS I'LL HAVE TO BE OK WITH BEING MEGA MAD AT YOU!

Yes, today I woke up ready to throw my crystal vase filled with "thinking of you" flowers across the room with the idea of slamming it against the wall to make an enormously loud sound, followed by shattering of glass into millions of pieces. That should make me feel better.

Today I woke up with the thought of punching someone (yes, even You) with such force my fist would ache, pain would be shared, and purple bruises would appear. That should make me feel better.

Today I woke up raring to scream at the top of my lungs and not just in the privacy of my closed closet. No intention of being prim, proper, or guarded. I wanted the entire world to hear. That should make me feel better.

Today I washed and changed sheets. As I forced them to fit the twin-size hospital mattress, the brand-new brown fitted sheet tore on two out of four corners, taking my fingernail with it. Pain, yells, colorful adult words.

Today I believe the wheelchair expanded an inch or two on each side overnight because it wouldn't fit through the bedroom door. I turned it frontwards. I turned it backwards. I tried to slide it in at an angle. Then, You saw me as I took a running start and rammed the swollen wheelchair against the frame. Success. The frame is now skinned with scalloped edging, but now that I think about it, I feel better... until I don't.

Guilt! Self-loathing. Self-hate. Self-disgust. *Guilt!* Why can't I just have a good old-fashioned temper tantrum without the aftermath of regret? I guess because I'm not alone. Jack is with me, experiencing my rage, frustration, anger, resentment, and pain. He pats me on the back and says, "It's okay, baby." I cry. Hug him. Pray silently. Ask forgiveness from Jack. I ask forgiveness from You, even though I know You understand.

We all love each other and we're in this together until the end and the new beginning. I'm still mad. There is a glimpse of "feel better" surfacing. Thank GOD!

I'm supposed to make life the best for Jack and then times like this happen and he comforts me. Go figure! Go guilt! I still *hate* this disease. I love Jack. I love You.

Thanks for loving me even when I'm mega mad at You.

Feeling Much Better,
LOVING YOU, AND JACK
Forever and a Day,
Debby

Be merciful to me, O God, be merciful to me!
For my soul trusts in you;
and in the shadow of your wings I will make my refuge,
until these calamities have passed by.
—Psalm 57:1

I can thank Him with my lips until . . .
I can thank Him with my heart.
—Dr. Charles Stanley

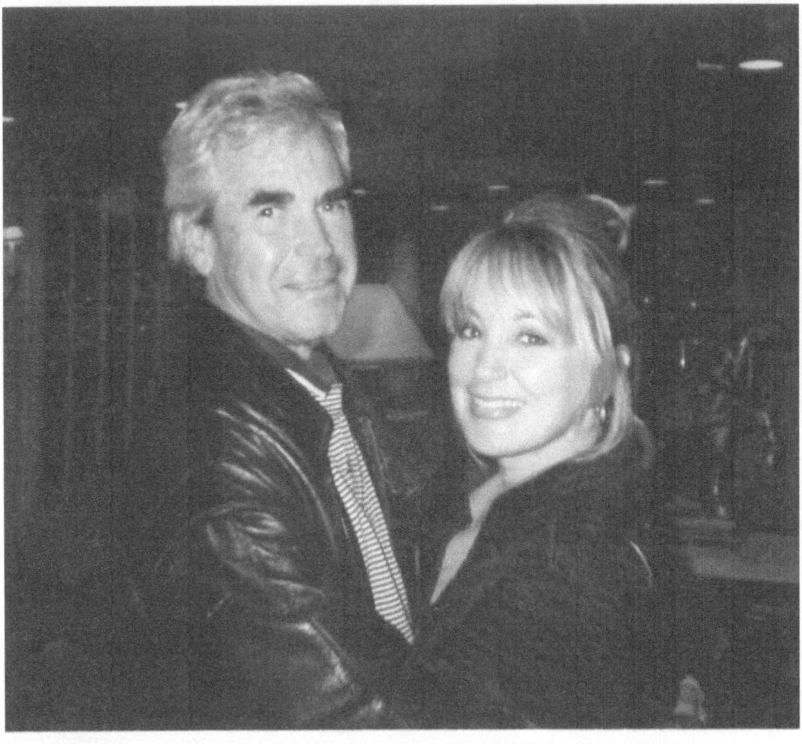

Mega Meltdown

Good morning, God!

Yesterday I had a meltdown with a capital M!

Linda, our friend and caregiver, came to the house to visit with Jack for a couple of hours so I could run a few errands. I hadn't even made it to the car before the tears began to flow. I hurried, buckled up, and pulled out of the neighborhood. I began to drive, think, and cry.

Pain. Brokenness. Grief. I told You I honestly wanted to die. Not figuratively, literally. I cried to You and pleaded with You to "Let me die!" The thoughts running through my head, my mind, my entire being, were frightening and dark. How, when, where? Next, I was praying for healing and forgiveness for the depression grabbing and crushing my spirit. Fear gripped my soul. Devastating ideas kidnapped my hope. What if You didn't come to my rescue? I drove aimlessly down the streets of my city, not knowing where to go, not caring where I went. I couldn't go home, not yet, not 'til I could get a grip! I felt unwanted, forgotten, desperate, alone, and hopeless. I honestly *didn't* want to die. I just wanted to remember how to be happy, to be loved, to be alive.

I made it home in new and improved shape. My cure? Turning up the contemporary Christian station with a few country renditions thrown in the mix, singing between sobs and other strange noises switched the channel in my mind. A glimmer of light. I feel tears in my eyes as I write these words, so I guess they are still pretty close to the surface.

I believe the main reason these feelings came with a vengeance was due to continuous, unrelenting fatigue and isolation. Only You and other caregivers of loved ones know what I'm speaking about. Those caregivers I do not know, however they know me, they know how I feel.

Please help me sort this out. What I should and shouldn't do in order to banish this cloud of darkness over my heart, soul, and mind. My precious husband needs me to be present, patient, loving, kind, capable, and strong. I'm searching, but feel only a faint spark left inside my being. Please ignite the light I'm losing before it is totally extinguished. The light of You. I know You will come to my rescue.

I LOVE YOU LORD.

All my love,
Forever and a Day,
Debby

I am the Light of the World. Whoever follows me will never walk in darkness, but will have the light of life.

—JOHN 8:12

Waiting with hope is very difficult, but true patience is expressed when we must even wait for hope. I will have reached the point of greatest strength once I have learned to wait for hope.

—GEORGE MATHESON

Alone-Lonely

Good morning, God!

I've been awake since 3:19 a.m. It's 5:28 now.
Being alone can be so lonely.
I've always loved my "alone time," but loneliness is totally different.
I'm alone. I'm lonely.
I tried to locate You this morning, but guess You're sleeping in, or solving some crisis in this or another universe.
Loneliness is a deep dark place where I know my heart is "in there" somewhere but I just can't find or feel it. And tucked behind the heart are my feelings of sadness, fear, despair, and numbness.
At the moment, all my tears are dried up. I've been crying too much lately, and I honestly don't know what or how to stop the flood of tears. Doesn't matter where I am or what I am doing, I start crying or sobbing at the drop of a hat.
I feel blank inside, like nothing is inside my being, just a crushed, broken soul, a bird with wounded wings, unable to take flight, a soul that has forgotten how to live, or laugh, or dream.
I'm going to stop, sit, be still, read my Bible, and my favorite scriptures. I pray that does the trick. Something has got to give. I am trusting the Holy Spirit is awake, and can revive this sleeping, despondent soul of mine.
To say depression has taken over is an understatement. I've dealt with this in the past, and I will trust You, Jesus, and the Holy Spirit to

bring me back from this darkness. "Even the dark- ness hides nothing from You. And with Your hand, You will guide me."

Please hurry Lord,
I truly need You.
Forever and a Day,
Debby

Fear and trembling have come upon me;
horror and fright have overwhelmed me.
And I say, oh, that I had wings like a dove!
I would fly away and be at rest.
—PSALM 55:5–6

Where can I go from your Spirit?
Where can I flee from your presence?
If I go up to the heavens, you are there;
if I make my bed in the depths, you are there.
If I rise on the wings of dawn,
if I settle on the far side of the sea,
even there your hand will guide me,
your right hand will hold me fast.
—PSALM 139:7–10

Friends

Good morning, God!

During our walk with Parkinson's and Lewy Body Dementia, friends come and go. Some stay awhile. Others check in on us frequently. Others are uncomfortable with the situation and move on. Our lives move on, also. Many times, we feel the sting. Ignored. Overlooked. Left behind. Shunned. Tolerated. Many more times we feel the joy. *Loved. Included. Cherished. Hugged. Pampered.*

Most friends and acquaintances don't and can't understand this disease. How can I expect them to understand? I've scoured, searched, and studied every scrap of information I could capture from books, magazines, physicians, support groups, symposiums, nurses, pamphlets, websites, and blogs. I don't and can't understand this disease either, and I am "the expert." The symptoms are listed in booklets. Nice, neat, and orderly. So ironic and so contradictory.

One constant that continues to resonate with me is that *every individual* walks their own unique path. Same diagnosis, same remarkable disease yet no experience is the same. *Beautiful minds. Beautiful people.*

Thank You for the gift of friendship in all its forms. People You place in our lives to lift our spirits, offer prayers, hugs, kisses, cards, phone calls, visits, and smiles.

Friends become strangers. Strangers become friends. New friends. Old friends. Family friends. Imaginary friends. Real friends! Thank You for Jack's "Candy Man!" Andy Mac! I never know when

"Mac" will show up. He seems to have a second sense for needed visits. Faithful. That's how I would describe Jack's best "in-town" friend. A knock at the door. I open it, and there stands Andy with a smile on his face, and an extra-large Hershey bar in his hand. He knows Jack! We hug. Andy proceeds to locate Jack, who is usually just around the corner perched in his geri-chair "watching" TV. I love to see the reaction between the two as Andy presents the perfect gift of chocolate, and says "Hey, Bird." The dark disease is lifted for a few minutes, and light walks into my hubby's broken spirit through the presence of a childhood friend. Smiles are exchanged. Jack "wakes up."

"Hey, Mac! How's your golf game?" Conversation begins.

Many times, the only words spoken by Jack are "Hey, Mac! How's your golf game?"

I see the true bond they share. Andy will sit with Jack in silence, or carry on a conversation by himself, one that describes their past experiences. "Remember the time . . ."

Childhood friends are discussed and mentioned by name and mischievous deeds. Laughter follows. A strange and wonderful sound . . . laughter.

Golf is always the beginning and the end of their conversation. Andy knows just how long to stay. He stands up, gives me a hug, shakes Jack's hand. Says, "See you later, Bird," and turns toward the front door. I see the pain in Andy's face. It's hard work being a best friend, especially at times such as these. Lately I've seen his hand reach for his face to wipe away a tear running down his cheek. I watch him as he walks across the street to his car. His head is looking down at the ground, shoulders bent just a bit. He'll be back. Even now, I believe Jack understands this blessing. This sacrifice. This gift.

Thank You for the "Candy Man."

He doesn't understand this remarkable disease.

He still knocks on our door. He still visits.

I love You Lord! I love Your friendship.
I love the people You have placed in our lives.
I love the friends You choose for us.
Forever and a Day,
Jack and Debby

If you see a friend without a smile, give him one of yours.
—PROVERB

No act of kindness, however small, is ever wasted.
—AESOP

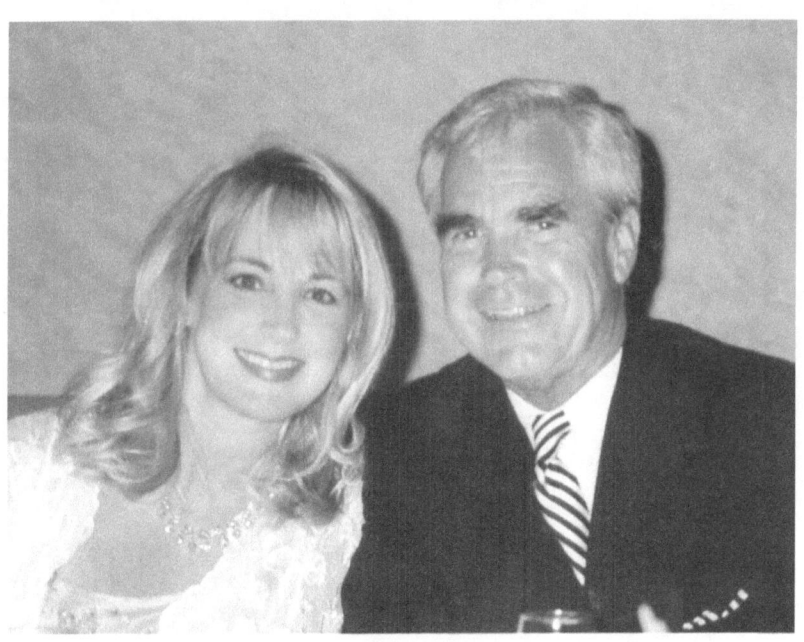

Oh, My Aching Back

Good morning, God!

How are You?

I know, You want to know how I'm doing . . . right? Let's just say—oh, my aching back.

I remember as a kid my mother would utter these words over and over again. "Oh, my aching back." I never knew what she was talking about. Well, now I can say I know.

Oh, my aching back, my aching leg, my aching bottom, and my aching arms.

Lifting, moving, arranging, rearranging. Lifts, wheelchairs, geri-chairs, pillows, blankets, headrests, household hospital beds, tiny unbendable husband, and everything in between is taking a major toll. My poor body is in critical condition.

Something else my mother would say that I had no way to relate to: "I'm no spring chicken." Well, now I can say I know that, too. I'm no spring chicken. I feel more like a plucked duck on its last leg.

Now that You know how I feel physically, could You please touch my body. Specifically, my *entire* left side. I need some serious relief. The day is still young and I'm not.

Thank goodness (and You) my spiritual self is in pretty good shape for the moment, or I would be cranking out some catchy, colorful, adult words dealing with this pain I'm carrying around.

My sense of humor and my spiritual self, tell me I can handle this, I'm a big girl now.

Big girls don't cry. Changed my mind. I'm not a big girl. I'm a little "old" lady. I do cry, and whine, and wince from this physical pain.

May I always praise You. No matter what aches in or on this awesomely wonderful body You gave me. Help me take better care of it. Better care of me.

Thanks for listening! You were listening. Weren't You?

Love You,
Forever and a Day
Debby

We have to love until it hurts.
It's not enough to say, "I love."
We must put that love into action.
And how can we do that?
By giving until it hurts.

—Mother Teresa

You made all the delicate, inner parts of my body,
and knit them together in my mother's womb.
Thank you for making me so wonderfully complex!
It is amazing to think about.

—Psalm 139:13–14

Struggles

God will use my struggles for good.
—Max Lucado

Good morning, God!

STRUGGLES!

I think of my own struggles, then put them aside to remember my sweet husband and his struggles.

I can't imagine.

He must depend on others for everything.

To feed, bathe, clothe, change, transport from bed to geri-chair and back again.

To speak for him, to anticipate and guess his requests.

To try to comfort him when we don't have a clue what is frightening him.

Why is he crying? What is he reaching for?

I hold his hand, stroke his arm, sit next to him, smooth his hair, kiss his cheek, rub his tummy, adjust his left leg (the one he hangs over the leg rest each and every day), and arrange his pillows so he doesn't fall to one side of the wheelchair.

Dinnertime is a new struggle, a different challenge for him and for us.

He needs reminders, encouragement, and coaxing.

He needs to be reminded to bite, to chew, and to swallow.

Everything I put on his plate is finger-food. Mashed potatoes and gravy, crawfish étouffée with rice, vanilla ice cream with hot fudge. It's *all* finger food.

After dinner I wipe his mouth of food and drool. He smiles at the touch of the warm cloth on his face. Chocolate dessert of some sort is his absolute favorite, so he has all he wants each night. Sippy cups are essential. He "helps" me guide the drink to his mouth. Many times, it's a battle, and we make a royal mess, but we get the job done.

Anyway, I'm sad for him and his struggles. Every minute of every day.

Of course, he is blessed to have me. "Sassy" kicks in every now and then.

I pray I honor my husband and his continuous struggles with the gift of Your love.

Even though these times are so difficult, I know when they are over, there is a part of me that will truly miss our struggles. I will miss "us." I've already missed us for so long now. I know I will also miss this part of our lives, as strange as that may sound.

Please use our struggles for good. Let us make a difference. As always, thanks for listening.

Forever and a Day,
My love,
Debby

I have carried you since you were born;
I have taken care of you from your birth.
Even when you are old, I will be the same.
Even when your hair has turned gray,
I will take care of you.
I made you and I will take care of you.
I will carry you and save you.

—ISAIAH 46:3–4

Quick Note

Good morning, God!

Monday! Again!
Just a quick note. I know You think I'm teasing. That I'll change my mind and write some lengthy "novel." But not today.
Just a quick note.
I love You to the moon and back!

Forever and a Day!
Debby

> *When I consider your heavens,*
> *the work of your fingers—*
> *the moon and the stars,*
> *which you have set in place—*
> *what is man that you are mindful of him?*
> —Psalm 8:3–4

> *I love You, Lord; you are my strength.*
> —Psalm 18:1

Basket Dreams

Good morning, God!

DREAMS?!?

I have my dreams in a medium-sized wicker basket tucked beside my bed.

Sometimes it makes me sad to glance at the "dream basket" but most of the time it gives me hope and makes me smile.

It's stuffed with clippings, magazines, notes, books, quotes, drawings, spiral notepads and all the ways "we're" going to make a difference. To make life happier. To give back. To comfort others. To create something marvelous.

I thought about moving my basket to the closet in the extra bedroom, so I don't have to look at it every other second. I waited a few minutes, then decided against it.

My dreams may not be going as planned, but at least I have them in plain sight. They remind me of the way You and I will change the world. They remind me that hope can come in the form of a medium-sized wicker basket nestled beside my nightstand.

I do believe You will help me to make some of these dreams come true—all for Your glory. I pray You will let me always dream, and hope, and create. That I will be able, through You, to comfort and help others by making their dreams come true through serving You.

Please grant me the discipline, perseverance, patience, imagination, and wisdom to help these dreams along the way to completion.

I love You Lord,
Forever and a Day,
Debby

P.S. Thank You for my dreams!

No eye has seen, no ear has heard,
no mind has conceived what God has prepared
for those who love him.
—1 CORINTHIANS 2:9

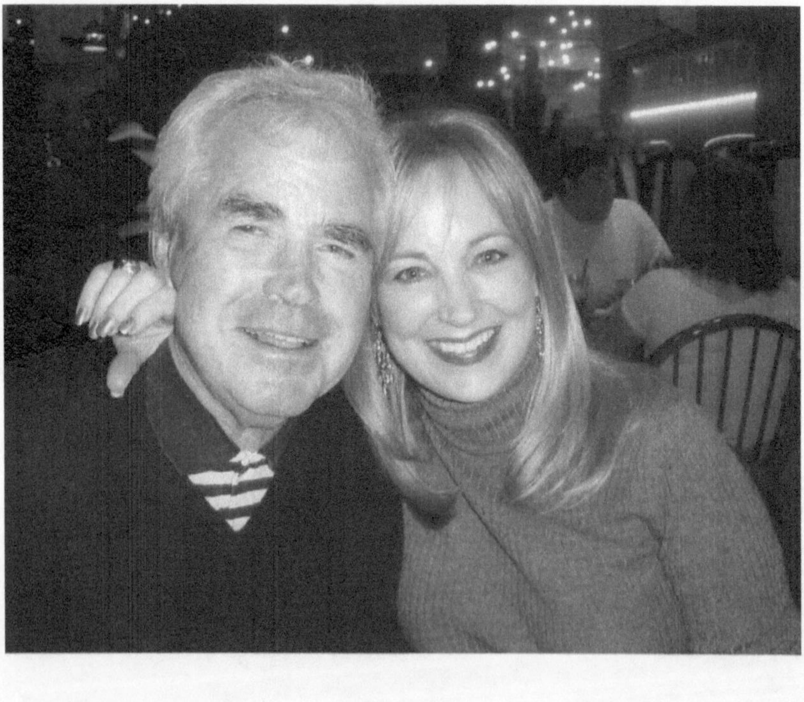

Praise Prayer

Good afternoon, God!

Thank You for a few miraculous gifts. My story begins yesterday on my way home from visiting my daughter. I was traveling seventy-seven miles an hour on Interstate 10 and I'd be home in thirty minutes. Cruising along, singing a song at the top of my voice, and You know I wasn't present the day You anointed those with beautiful, angelic vocal cords. I sing anyway, especially alone in the car, when it's just me and my music.

Next thing I knew, the car started making weird noises and veering to the right. I made it to an exit that would take me to familiar territory. I stopped at the nearest gas station.

The left rear tire was in shreds. Lovely! What a predicament. Linda was staying with Jack, so I called to let her know my situation. My son and the tow company came to my rescue. It was Sunday. Repair shop was closed. I made arrangements to leave my car overnight, so they can assess the damage and give me a call in the morning.

The tire center called the next day to let me know the situation, solution, and cost.

Four-hundred and sixty-six dollars! I needed two new tires! Remember how I've been struggling with faith and funds? My fear resurfaced instantly at the sound of the sweet, manly voice on the other end of the line. Fresh news of additional, unexpected, and unwelcome expenditures. Panic prayer or praise prayer. You tell me.

Okay. Going with praise prayer. However, my stomach is still queasy.

Later that morning I picked up my car, all decked out with two extra-shiny new tires.

Now, I could travel in safety if only I had money for gas. I know ... praise prayer.

On my way home, I stopped by the post office to pick up my mail. Amongst the nonsense mail, and monthly bills, there was a precious little hand-addressed envelope for me. I opened my little card and read the note. "This is what friends are for." If that wasn't enough, my friend had included a check for five-hundred dollars!

I cried in the post office, in my car, on the way to buy groceries, and on my drive home. Not little tiny tears. Giant, nonstop oceans of tears. When I arrived home, I called Terry to thank her for purchasing my new tires and You guessed it, I cried again.

You are awesome! I love the surprises and blessings You send our way, and the manner in which You deliver them.

After I calmed down, I was trying to understand the flood of tears. It came to me. It wasn't just the surprise of the money at the perfect time. Someone thought of us—my friend remembered me. She cared enough to take the time to write a sweet note. The generous check was a magnanimous act of kindness. She didn't know my situation, my insecurities, my fears. However, You did. Everything about this experience was incredible. A miracle.

Praise Prayer

Thank You for safety, family, tow trucks, repair shops, friends, new tires, and enough money left over for gas! You're the MAN!

I will praise Your name,
Forever and a Day,
Love, Debby

A CAREGIVER'S CONVERSATIONS WITH GOD

*Lord my God, you have done many miracles,
your plans for us are many.
If I tried to tell them all,
there would be too many to count.*
—PSALM 40:5

*You cannot do a kindness too soon,
for you never know how soon it will be too late.*
—RALPH WALDO EMERSON

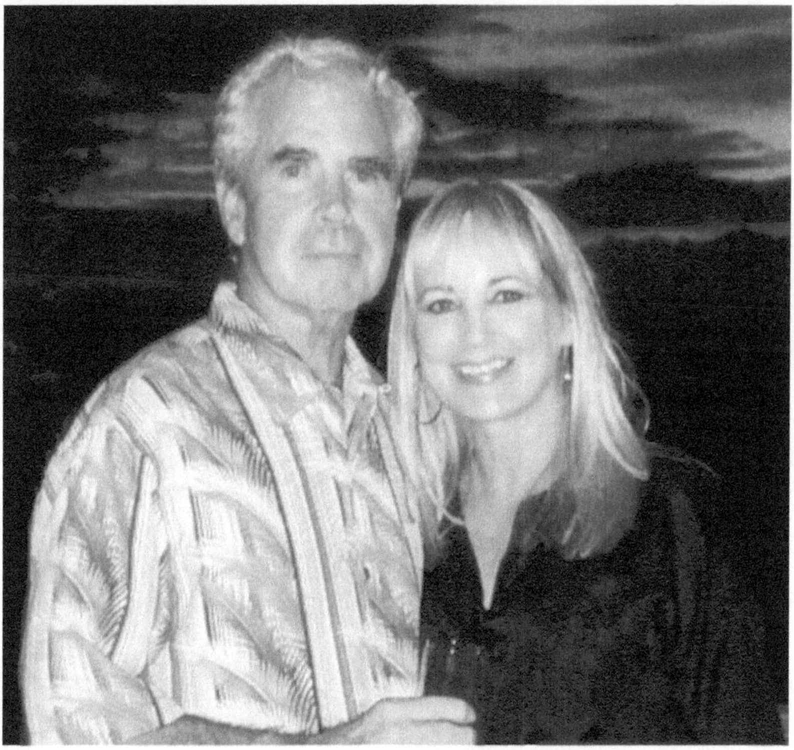

"The Day"

Good morning, God!

So much has happened since our last journal conversation.
I'm still numb. I'm still lost.
Jack came to be with You in heaven on Tuesday, October 14. His dad's birthday.
He had been nonresponsive all day Monday with labored, yet peaceful, rhythmic breathing.
I sat with him, held his hand, kissed his face, patted his chest, prayed our prayers. I took him down memory lane. Reliving our stories, our dates, our golf trips, and our family. I reminded him of the sweet things he would do and say. It was most definitely a tender day.
During the night, his breathing became more of a struggle. The hospice nurse had instructed me earlier in the day regarding the medicine I could administer that would calm his breathing. I gave it to him twice during the night, in small doses. Nurses assured me I wasn't in any way contributing to his death, only making him more comfortable. I struggled with this, but his breathing did calm and that was good.
I slept with him in his man cave and tiny twin-sized hospital bed Monday night. For four years his bed always seemed much too small. Monday and Tuesday the bed was entirely too enormous. I wanted to be closer to him, to have the bed be cozier, and yes, even smaller.
My head rested on his chest, with one hand placed to feel his

beating heart, the other hand to hold his. Our bodies cuddled so close there was no separation at all. Once again, we were "one." I tried to be brave, and strong. You know tears are necessary and always in abundance for this courageous "cry baby." Kleenex boxes surrounded me. Puddles of my tears rested on his LSU T-shirt. I sang songs that popped in my head, talked to let him know I was close (in case the weight of my body pressing on his wasn't sufficient). I whispered words of love, reassurance, and hope. I reminded him he was on his way to heaven and so many people he had cherished and treasured in this lifetime were anxiously awaiting his arrival. Open arms and open hearts.

My arms and heart, on the other hand, were wrapped around my sweet Jack. Someone would need to pry me from the gentle "death grip" I had on him.

Why did he have to go? Why couldn't he stay? Why didn't the miracle cure arrive?

Why didn't You, the Great Physician, heal him? Why couldn't I go with him?

Questions. Answers? Please!

Your presence during the last two days of our lives together will be remembered forever. I felt You with every breath I took. Thank You for spending those precious moments, hours, and days in his man cave, in that tiny twin bed with us. Peaceful, yet powerful. Thank You for taking Jack to his new heavenly home.

I'm jealous. I know You still have plans for me in this life, please stay with me. I desperately need You. Seems I'm struggling to breathe, to hope, to focus.

I'm numb. I'm lost. I know You will come to my rescue once again.

You are my "knight in shining armor," my comforter, counselor, provider, and best friend forever!

You'll have to excuse me, it's time to cry again. I'll talk to You later.

Please kiss Jack for me. Tell him I will always love him. Tell him I will miss him every minute of every day.

Tell him I will see him soon.

Forever and a Day,
My love for the two of you!
Debby

He will wipe away every tear from their eyes,
and there will be no more death or sorrow or crying or pain.
All these things will be gone forever.
—REVELATION 21:4

In my Father's house are many mansions;
if it were not so, I would have told you.
I go to prepare a place for you.
And if I go and prepare a place for you,
I will come again and receive you to myself;
that where I am, there you may be also.
—JOHN 14:2–3

Difficult Days

Good afternoon, God!

It's January 13.

It's the thirteenth of the month, and I have been upset all day . . . crying, sobbing, walking around aimlessly. I've asked myself, "What is your problem?" Then, I realize something astonishing. Mind-boggling. The difficult days of each month are the thirteenth through the seventeenth and it all began last October.

One beautiful October blue-sky day, I left the house to run errands. Post office, grocery store, pharmacy, and, hopefully, a walk at the park. I had an hour and a half before time to head back to the house and my sweet hubby. Linda was at the house with Jack. I had been gone approximately fifteen minutes when my phone rang, it was Linda. She called me Boss Lady no matter how many times I tried to coax her into calling me by my first name. I'll always remember where I was, the place, the time, the day, the exact spot in the parking lot of the post office. I heard the ring, noticed the name on caller ID, and frantically maneuvered my handbag and bundle of mail to answer my cell phone. I heard the voice on the other end of the line. "Boss Lady, you need to come home now. Doc isn't responding, it's time." I don't remember answering her. I don't remember hanging up. I do remember sitting in the car for a few minutes trying to comprehend the magnitude of her statement and what it encompassed. Fog covered my being and took over my physical movements without any direction from my mind. I backed out of the parking lot and slowly began to drive not the shortest route home. I drove around in circles for about ten minutes then I guess that's when my thoughts finally kicked in, and I decided I must go home to hold my dying husband. Time had caught up with us, and the remaining moments were precious. I gathered my composure, wiped the tears and makeup staining my face, and found my way home.

The thirteenth through the seventeenth of each month are difficult days. I am present. I am absent. I am numb. I am lost. I am sad.

The day of waiting. The day of saying goodbye. The day of dying. The day of celebrating Jack's life. The day of holding my family. These days sneak up on me.

I wonder, "Why am I so sad?" I was doing pretty well, then the calendar reminded me what my heart already knows.

Our last days. Our last touch. Our last hug. Our last kiss. Then I understand. Sadness makes sense.

I'm ready to be happy during those days. Surely they'll come, won't they?

I Love You Lord,
Forever and a Day,
Debby

We didn't lose the game; we just ran out of time.
—Vince Lombardi

He will once again fill your mouth with laughter
and your lips with shouts of joy.
—Job 8:21

Valentine's Celebration

Good afternoon, God!

It's rainy and Louisiana's version of cold: wet and forty degrees.

I just got home from the grocery. A few basics were needed for the "blizzard."

I was walking down the Valentine's Day gift aisle, and for a second I thought, "Oh, I need to get a card and something in the form of milk chocolate for Jack." Then I smiled, then I fought back the tears, then I started remembering Valentine's Days of the past.

One year, early in our relationship, Jack waited 'til the last possible minute to make dinner reservations. Yes, that was his assignment. "Southern gentleman" is a title he wore proudly. After calling all our favorite places in town, and doing "drive-bys", we eventually decided to eat Popeyes Fried Chicken in the comfort of our own home. I was a tad disappointed (hysterical crying, sulking, feeling unappreciated, on and on). A Valentine's Day meltdown is always so attractive.

After the sanity returned to our love nest, we decided to celebrate Valentine's Day every February 15. That way we would be reminded on the 14th that the 15th was right around the corner. We would not have to hurry in order to wait to be seated at an overcrowded, understaffed, pricey, noisy restaurant. Not to mention what a splendid deal on cards, chocolates, and SweeTart sweethearts. Probably half price. Our official Valentine's Day was changed to February 15.

I loved that about us. We would make our own rules if we felt it necessary, and as the years went by, there were many occasions new rules were definitely needed. But, we liked romance, and we loved each other, so we always made it happen.

We kept all our cards. Our treasures of keepsakes. We have beautiful wooden boxes filled with Valentine love notes. I've decided that's the gift I'll treat myself to this year. I'll pour myself a glass (or two) of chardonnay, have a piece (or four) of chocolate, toast our day and enjoy rereading the cards we chose for each other every year. I love to see his handwriting. I know I will trace his "I love you, Jack" with my index finger, close the card, and hold it close to my heart, then gently set it aside and open the next.

I have my date planned, my reservation in place. Popeyes Fried Chicken sounds like the perfect entree. Can't wait.

Forever and a Day,
Our Love for Each Other,
Our Love for You,
Jack and Debby

"*I walk down memory lane because I love running into you.*"

Every time I think of you, I give thanks to my God.
—Philippians 1:3

Wheels

Good morning, God!

Wheelchairs! I've seen two today. Each one brought a sadness over memories of "us," and for those I saw today walking the road we just completed.

I'm downtown at a local coffee shop, having a cup of Moroccan mint hot tea. I dropped the car off at the shop and walked the block and a half to the Stellar and Bean Coffee Shop and waited for the brakes and brake fluid to be checked. The blinding red light keeps flashing to let me know my car needs attention. So, after much procrastination, I finally dropped my car off at the shop. The car repairs weren't the main topic of conversation, Jack was. Everyone in town knew, loved, and respected Jack. Sweet, rugged mechanics in greasy name-tagged shirts and matching deep blue trousers gave me hugs and condolences. Mechanics who worked on Jack's parade of cars for decades. They told me how wonderful Dr. Worley was, and that he was in a better place. The facial expressions and tender actions of those burly guys touched my heart with their genuine display of love and loss.

Between the wheelchairs and the conversation about Jack, I'm emotionally taxed. Sometimes it doesn't take much for this munchkin. Thus, the strong cup of exotic tea.

I've been looking at potential directions for my new life. That's not accurate. It's really not my new life, it's just a new phase, a new chapter. A brand-new adventure I hadn't planned to take by myself.

I'm proud to say I've made progress. I'm still running around in circles, just not so fast and furious. Yes, that's how I define progress at the moment: a slower circle running.

I'm narrowing my options. Accessing my assets. Reviewing my finances. Remembering my passions. I've made a few connections, met with friends and advisors. I'm surrounding myself with people who dream, encourage, uplift, laugh, hug, and make me excited I actually crawled out of bed.

I know You will guide me. Please continue to open doors and close windows (so I won't be tempted to jump). May my life unfold into something beautiful for You.

Thank You that our lives don't include wheelchairs or walkers or geri-chairs. I realize in some strange way I really do miss those "helpers", our "wheels", our "vehicles," because I miss Jack. I miss us. However, I know Jack is healed and I'm working on myself.

A text just notified me, "Your car is ready to go." Time to finish my cup of Moroccan mint tea. The warmth of the tea should stay with me as I walk the block and a half to the repair shop, although cool air sounds inviting and invigorating.

I do pray You will bless those I saw today pushing their loved ones in their wheelchairs, all bundled up in blankets, hats, and gloves. The look on their faces said it all. I remember those feelings of putting one foot in front of the other. Please send people into their lives to brighten their way and lighten their hearts.

Forever and a Day,
My love for You,
Debby

P.S. Thanks for wheels, repair-shop friends, hot tea, and quality time with You.

*For I know the plans I have for you, declares the Lord,
plans to prosper you and not harm you,
plans to give you hope and a future.*
—Jeremiah 29:11

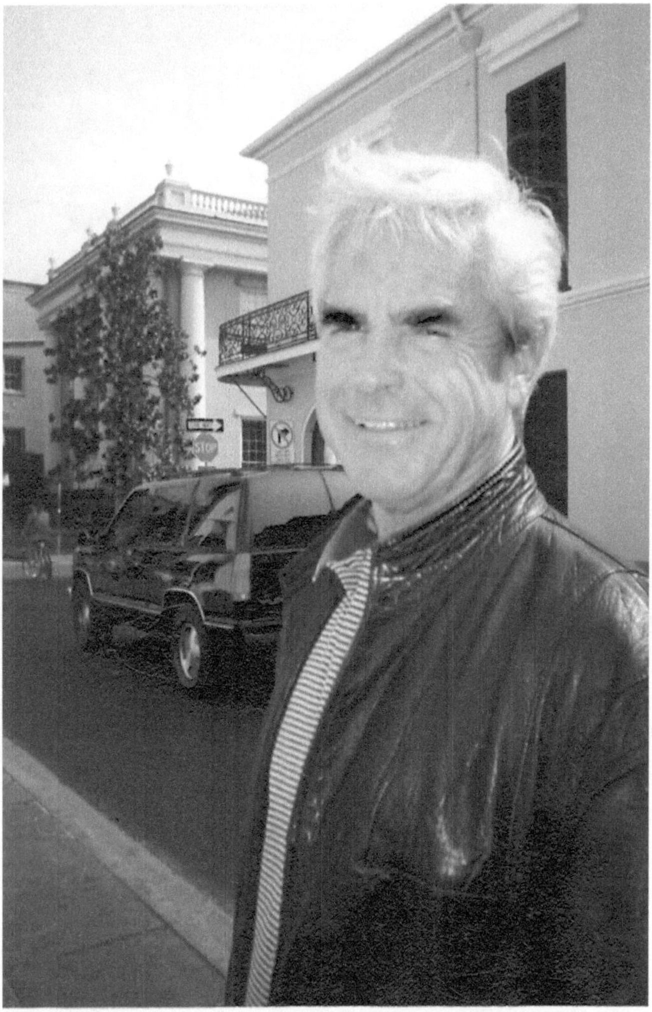

Holding Hands

Good morning, God!

I wish I had a hand to hold. Right now, right this minute!

I keep looking at my hands, trying to remember what it feels like for someone I love to hold them. I've tried on several occasions to hold my own hand, and it never, ever works.

I miss holding my grandparents' hands plus their bear hugs, so tight I thought my heart was going to pop right out of my chest.

I miss holding my parents' hands, when I was a little girl skipping to school with my lunch box in one hand and Mom's hand in the other.

I miss holding my children's hands, since they are miles away, with little hands of their own to hold now.

I miss holding my husband's hands, because he's in heaven, holding Yours.

Jack and I were the champions of hand holding. It was so natural, even from the beginning of our relationship. Until his last breath and beyond, we held hands.

Disease had taken away many activities we enjoyed as a couple. Hand-holding remained a constant until death took Jack away and even then, the memories remain. I can close my eyes and see us walking hand in hand. Friends would give us a hard time. They accused us of acting like a couple of teenagers. Guilty as charged! We told each other they were just jealous. Their comments didn't interfere with the oneness we shared with the mere touch of each other's hands. So simple, yet so comforting, so magical, so healing. So much love shared, just by taking someone's hand.

So, watch out world, it's my mission to do some serious hand holding today. Place a tiny bottle of hand sanitizer in your bag if you must and be on the lookout for a petite blonde about 5'4" (if she's wearing her stiletto wedges). That will be me, reaching out to hold your hand and share a little love.

You talk about holding hands in Your Scriptures. "I am the Lord Your God, Who holds your right hand."

Let me remember to reach out and hold someone's hand today. Thank you for reminding me that You are always holding mine.

Forever and a Day,
Debby

I am the Lord your God,
who holds your right hand, and I tell you,
"Don't be afraid. I will help you."
—Isaiah 41:13

Heavenly Majesty

Good morning, God!

Thank You for Your gift of the heavens. Sunrise, sunset, clouds, sun, moon, stars. Colors. Rainbows. I'm learning to gaze, and many times *stare* at Your glorious heavens. They give me comfort, make me smile, lift my spirit, wrap me up in a soft blanket covered in love.

Not long ago, I wasn't feeling much love from You . . . or anyone else for that matter. I was sad, pitiful, with my head hung low or looking straight ahead and really not enjoying the scenery. Then it happened. You happened, Your voice happened. The whisper told me to "look up." I looked up, in the darkest time of my life, one of the darkest nights, to a heaven so magnificently magical, stunning, and holy! Tears started rolling down my cheeks. I couldn't take my eyes away from the perfect beauty of Your masterpiece. Your love spread across a velvety black sky covered in twinkling, dancing, brilliant white stars. Just to the side, the sliver of the moon. Even the darkness hides nothing from You. You make even the darkness beautiful when it is touched by Your hand.

So, when I'm happy, when I'm sad, when I'm lonely, when I miss Jack, when I miss You, I have a place I visit: Your heavens. I look up. I tell You I love You. I tell Jack I miss him. I tell you both good night and sweet dreams.

Your daytime heavens can be just as magnificent, but at this point in my life, the night is the brightest!

Please tell Jack good night and give him a kiss for me!

Love You,
Forever and a Day,
Debby

The heavens tell the glory of God,
and the skies announce what his hands have made.
Day after day they tell the story;
night after night they tell it again.
They have no speech or words;
they have no voice to be heard.
But their message goes out through all the world;
their words go everywhere on earth.

—P<small>SALM</small> 19:1–4

He determines the number of the stars
and calls them each by name.

—P<small>SALM</small> 147:4

Doors – Thresholds

Good evening, God!

Today I found these "feeling" notes tucked in my journal. In a previous entry I'd written about the *facts* the day You came to take Jack to his heavenly home and the months that followed. The words on this page describe my heart's unspeakable aching and longing that took place on "The Day." Healing continues. You and Jack are constantly on my mind. I'm moving forward most days . . . we won't mention the "other" days. I have made a daring, decisive decision to open the door of my heart so I can mend more completely. I know scars will remain . . . engraved and cherished. Doors will be opened. Thresholds will be crossed. *Today!*

"The Day"— Heart Thoughts

Good morning God!

I stand at the door to Jack's "man cave." Silence is all I hear. I tell myself, "Don't step over, don't step in, because then death will be real, and we can't go back." So, I just stand at the door, frozen except for the heat of my coffee cup cradled in both hands. Please God, just one more cup of coffee, then he can go. I promise. Jack's not breathing. Neither am I for a moment, a moment that seems like an eternity. Then, I take a deep breath and think maybe I can breathe for both of us.

Again, I tell myself it won't be true, it won't be real, it won't count, unless I cross the threshold. Once I walk through the door into Jack's man cave, only then will death be real. So, I just stand and stare, completely frozen.

The threshold to accepting death. Accepting new life. Accepting raw reality. Accepting what I see. Accepting what I know, I know.

Jack's doorway.

Jack's door—opening, shutting, closing, closed. People take him away.

Strangers take his hospital bed, his meds, his supplies, his nurses, his doctors. The room is empty now. There are scars, nicks, and gouges on the frame of the door from the wheelchair straining to fit through the tiny opening to the room. Jack and I share similar scars, nicks, and gouges from this journey we traveled together.

Five Months and Counting

I still have trouble knowing whether to open or shut the door. The room is different, not a man cave anymore, more of a guest room, needing some repairs and a fresh coat of color. Rainbow colors. That's probably what Jack is enjoying about now.

Minutes, hours, days, months. The door. The threshold. The crossing. So much has happened, but time continues to stand still in many ways.

Thank You for taking Jack's hand and leading him to his mansion! He so deserves the mansion You prepared for him.

I'm trying my best to move forward, to make some kind of progress. I've tried to rush this process . . . to hurry and finish this phase. When that doesn't work, I try to make myself slow down to take care of myself. So, I'm back and forth, in and out of the doorway—the threshold—the crossing.

Miracle of Miracles

This morning I chose to be brave. I threw open all the doors. I'm welcoming new life.

The beauty of living nudges me to cross the threshold. Please take my hand, too, and walk with me as I step into the future.

Love You and Jack,
Forever and a Day,
Debby

The pain passes, but the beauty remains.
—Pierre-Auguste Renoir

When one door of happiness closes, another opens;
but often we look so long at the closed door
that we do not see the one which has been opened for us.
—Helen Keller

My "Selves"

Good morning, God!

It's 7:01 a.m. Monday morning, and my "bossy self" has been yelling and nagging at me even before I got out of bed.

So many "selves", so many versions of myself harassing me and giving me orders, suggestions, demands, and reprimands.

Then my "nurturing self" comes to my defense and reminds me I need rest and to take care of myself, telling me *that's more like it*. I love my "nurturing self" but then she ruins it all by telling me to exercise just when I thought she was my best friend.

Then there's my "sad self," my "lazy self," my "crazy self," and my "I-don't-know-what-to-do-with-the-rest-of-my-life-without-Jack self." Multiple personalities . . . how many can a girl be blessed with? Grief seems to unleash a multitude.

Grieving isn't what I thought it would be at all!

It's strenuous work. It's grueling, relentless, and unpredictable. I guess I thought it would be a gradual, steady climb upward from sadness and crying to smiles, laughter, sweet memories. One morning I would wake up to find my "happy self" once again.

My dad always said I was a dreamer. Well, my version of grieving was totally a fairy-tale version of the true process.

Just when I think I'm fine and doing a great job, my "crazy self" appears and assures me I am one of the "wackiest chicks" on Your planet.

So, here I am asking for Your help. Please help me to discover a more balanced self today. Please calm my many "selves." Help me in my climb, in my grieving. When I become overwhelmed with voices racing around in my head, I will trust You and Your wisdom, directions, suggestions. Your Voice.

Thank You for Your beautifully calming whispers. I feel so much better! How about You?

All my love,
Forever and a Day!
Debby

Trust in the Lord with all your heart
and lean not on your own understanding;
in all your ways acknowledge him,
and he will direct your paths.
—PROVERBS 3:5–6

Be still and know that I am God.
—PSALM 46:10

Wedding Anniversary

Good morning, God!

I did it! With a little help from You.

I made it quite nicely through the first wedding anniversary day without Jack here to celebrate with me.

"Nicely" is a unique way to describe my emotions but, in a strange way, that word fits perfectly.

I felt close to Jack all day long. I turned the music on while I organized, wrote, cleaned, and huddled at home with my memories, and pictures of our wedding day. We were so pretty. Yes, pretty is the way I describe Jack. So pretty! Hollywood Handsome. There were occasions during the day when I started to focus too much on "us." I would dance, or sing, or clean to keep myself from boo-hooing. Success was mine. I made it!

You and Jack had already planned a special evening for me with four of my craziest friends. Paula called Monday and said we were going to have a "girls' night." "Night" indicates 5:00 to 7:30 and "girls" indicates wishful thinking. When I hung up the phone to jot down the information in my calendar, I did one of those smile-cry faces. I saw the date. March 5! Our anniversary! Three of the four friends that I celebrated with have lost their husbands within the last two years; the other has been married to her high school sweetheart for forty-seven years. The company was a perfect gift. We put the *girl* back in girlfriends.

Thank you for planning a special evening for me.

I miss you, Jack. I bet your ears were ringing. We talked a lot about you, about us, about our friends. All good stuff. I often wonder what you are doing in heaven. I talk to you, I look up at the sky and wave to you when I'm in the backyard. You know how crazy I am. Hopefully the neighbors don't know yet. The gesture makes me feel closer to you. Thank you for all the years of wonderful, romantic anniversary celebrations. They were the best! Just like my Hollywood Handsome husband.

Kudos to You, dear God, for letting me share such special moments and memories with this amazing man. Kisses and hugs to both of you.

Thanks for fresh old memories and good old friends.
Forever and a Day,
Debby

I will praise you, Lord, with all my heart;
I will tell of all the marvelous things you have done.
I will be filled with joy because of you.
I will sing praises to your name, O Most High.

—Psalm 9:1–2

We've Already Spoken

Good morning, God?

We've already spoken this morning for quite a while and for this I am truly sorry! Sorry for the tears, the panic, the fear.

You've helped me calm down, my heart is beating with a steady beat, and my craziness has subsided.

Thank You for everything.

Please speak to me today. Guide me in the way I should go. I'm confused and need added direction. Should I wait for You? Should I step out in faith? Should I do both? And, how exactly does that look??

Please open my eyes, my ears, and my heart. Open them to Your ways, and Your voice.

I desperately need You every moment of my life and this is definitely one of those moments.

Love You,
Forever and a Day,
Debby

God is not a God of confusion, but a God of peace.
—1 Corinthians 14:33

Let the morning bring me word of your unfailing love,
for I have put my trust in you.
Show me the way I should go, for to you I lift up my soul.
—Psalm 143:8

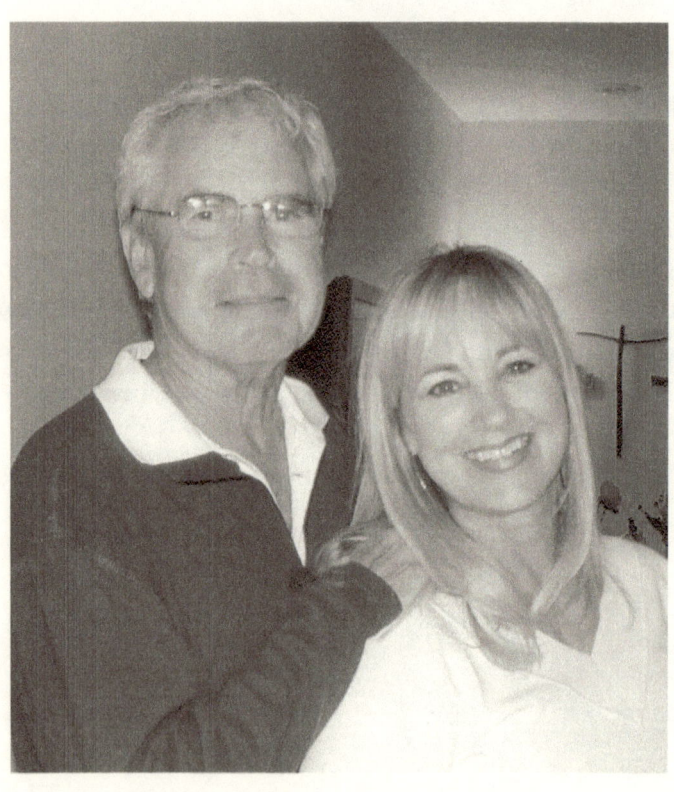

Smiles and Laughter

Good morning, God!

I smiled and laughed yesterday. Whether I wanted to or not. And I'm happy to report, I wanted to.

Today I am thankful I'm learning to cry in more appropriate settings and situations. For the past five-and-a-half months, I have had no earthly or heavenly control over my tears. Some of my most "memorable" episodes take place in the grocery store, on any aisle, at any time. The background elevator music playing golden oldies only intensifies the melancholy. Another example of inappropriate behavior took place standing in line at the Department of Motor Vehicles. A simple task for the day to renew my driver's license. You guessed correctly, streams of silent tears rolling down my face and dripping off my chin. Disturbing myself and making others feel uncomfortable. Total strangers staring at me, wondering whether to hug me or call a nice policeman to escort me from the building to a facility for the fragile.

Today, I am also thankful I don't cry as often, or as long, or as much.

I know You're happy about that because You're the One who is my designated cry catcher. Sorry! However, You have done an excellent job, and You do possess awfully big shoulders, and yes, You should receive some sort of award.

In conclusion, I guess I'm happy I'm smiling more, and I'm happy I'm crying less! Jack always told me, "It doesn't take much to entertain you."

Jack was right back then, and now that he's in heaven with You I believe I can hear his words again.

I've always loved life, loved to laugh, loved to love and loved to feel. I believe I may just have to shed a few tiny tears to celebrate this big fat smile I have spread across my lovely face.

Anyway, another day of concentrated progress. At some point I expect my feelings and my progress will be more automatic. But, it's okay if I need a little gentle push from me to me and from You to me! Thanks for all the times You sit with me while I cry and the times You laugh with me and the times You can see me in the future, knowing I'm smiling and filled with hope.

As always, please give Jack my love!

Forever and a Day,
Debby

Start every day with a smile, and get it over with.
—W. C. Fields

Laughter is the shortest distance between two people.
—Victor Borge

Laughter is the sun that drives winter from the human face.
—Victor Hugo

Where is My "Want to?"

Good morning, God!

Where is my "want to?"

If I see it or feel it, it's just in tiny spurts, then magically disappears. Much like walking toward a mirage, only to find it's a figment of my imagination.

I want to want to . . . but I don't.

At this moment, I want to sit in this uncomfortable chair the rest of my life!

At this moment I *don't* want to sit in this uncomfortable chair the rest of my life!

Please help me get up and get on with my life. Why is it so difficult?

My prayer today is for the gumption to get up and move. Please show me which way to go, to the right or to the left.

Please walk with me. Please whisper, "This way, this is the way you should go, this is the way for you. I'll be with you. I'll never leave you. I'll never forget you. I'll never forsake you. I'll hold your right hand, so don't be afraid."

I still don't really want to, but I'm going to get up from this uncomfortable chair. As long as I can picture You by my side, who knows, maybe a miracle might just happen. I may reconnect with my long-lost friend—my "want to."

> I Love You Lord, Forever and a Day,
> Debby

If you go the wrong way
— to the right or to the left—
you will hear a voice behind you saying,
"This is the right way. You should go this way."
—Isaiah 30:21

The Lord says, "I will guide you
along the best pathway for your life.
I will advise you and watch over you."
—Isaiah 32:8

Mountain Worship

Good morning, God!

Thank You I don't have to climb to the tip-top of a mighty mountain to find You. Let's face it and be totally honest: I have extremely short little legs, and my strides are nothing to brag about. I haven't exercised on a regular basis in about seven years (sad, but true). I start breathing heavily walking the aisles of our local grocery store. So, mountain climbing is not achievable at this time in my life. Doesn't sound exciting, anyway. Wears me out just anticipating the attempt.

The last few years have taken a toll on my once gorgeous, toned, muscular body. I tend to exaggerate on occasion. However, adding twenty pounds, accompanied by insufficient exercise, is not a pretty picture.

There is an overgrown grassy knoll in my ten-by-twelve-foot backyard that I could "climb" if necessary. I would do that to talk to You if required. I'm just so grateful I don't have to climb mountains or grassy knolls to worship You.

I know I sound a wee bit dramatic, but I *really* am thankful I can pray, talk, visit, sing, and worship You no matter where I am, and I do, beginning before I climb out of bed each morning. I will start the drudgery of molding my body back into recognizable shape. I know that is important, because that's where the Holy Spirit resides. Poor thing.

Thank You so much for the Holy Spirit and Your presence. May I always worship You in holiness, reverence, and awe.

Love You . . .
Forever and a Day,
Debby

"You will search for me.
And when you search for me with your whole heart,
you will find me!
I will let you find me," says the Lord.
—JEREMIAH 29:13

The Little Magnolia Tree

Good morning, God!

    The little magnolia tree in the front yard is beginning to bloom. My heart smiles a sad smile with cherished memories.
    I go back in time and remember the days I would be standing at the kitchen sink preparing our "after golf" dinner, and Jack would sneak up behind me and, by magic, a perfectly beautiful magnolia blossom would appear in front of me.
    Jack would smile like a little boy presenting an extravagant gift to his girlfriend. I'm so happy I was his "princess." He would insist I put it in water in a crystal vase on the windowsill *immediately* but only after he pulled me close and gave me soft love kisses.
    I can't begin to remember how many times Jack walked through the front door with his treasures. I do know I will never forget such simple, yet elegant gifts of love.
    Thank You for magnolias, kisses, hugs, and love.

Forever and a Day,
Debby

Love is the beauty of the soul—
—St. Augustine

I Love You Roses

Good morning, God!

Thank you for the little surprises You send my way.

This morning I've been going through stored boxes in the garage. I have books, and books, and more books.

All shapes, sizes, types, beautiful, historical, informative, inspirational and on and on.

I came across a very special book, *Lucky Man,* by Michael J. Fox, our hero, advocate, and unknown friend.

As I opened the pages, I found a pressed faded white rose.

Guess I had tucked it between the pages many years ago.

The first time Jack sent me white roses, I thanked him for my beautiful white "I Love You" roses. He loved the title I had given them, thus their coronation. From that day forward, it's been their official name.

A sweet memory of the way Jack used to show his love to me—white "I Love You Roses." Sometimes bouquets, sometimes dozens, sometimes just a single-stemmed white rose.

Every now and then, I happen upon these wonderful surprises that remind me of Jack's *forever love,* and I am allowed to feel his presence once again.

Forever and a Day,
Debby

*Love is like a rose.
When pressed between two lifetimes,
it will last forever.*
—AUTHOR UNKNOWN

Jack's Two-Dollar Bill

Good morning, God!

Remember the $2.00 bill?

The one Jack carried in his pocket all the time for all those years? For luck.

The one "DD" had given him. Diane, his baby "sissy." She called him "Bubby."

Jack never requested presents for birthdays, Father's Day, or anniversaries, however he always secretly loved them and wanted to receive gifts wrapped in beautiful packages with pretty bows. The more plentiful, the bigger his smile.

I don't know the complete story about the $2.00 bill. I do know it was a gift from his grown-up baby sister. He said he would never, under any circumstances, spend it, with the implication "don't touch my stuff."

Diane was ten years younger than Jack. In many ways, I believe the age difference made their relationship stronger. Jack cherished the paper bill and carried it with him in his back pocket every day for decades.

Over the years the paper, once crisp with that new smell of money, became faded, wrinkled, bent, torn, and taped. The green was worn, and most wouldn't recognize the paper as currency of any kind. Nonetheless, it was still carried and treasured, tucked in "Bubby's" back pocket.

When Jack went to heaven, I put all his personal pocket items in a special wooden box. One thing was missing. The $2.00 bill. I searched everywhere, with no luck. You must have seen my weariness and sadness over Jack's treasure. It was as if I had lost another part of my ruggedly handsome husband. A few weeks later, I received change from a purchase I made. The change included a couple of twenties and a crisp new $2.00 bill!

I know without a doubt that You and Jack sent some love my way. The new bill is once again tucked in a safe place.

If I live long enough, I'll become like the $2.00 bill. Faded, wrinkled, torn, and taped.

I'm just fine with that, because I know I'm safely tucked in Your back pocket.

Thank You.

Thank You for making Jack brand-new and crisp!

Thank You for "DD" and the unique and precious $2.00 gift.

Forever and a Day,
My love for You,
Debby

For where your treasure is, there will your heart be also.
—MATTHEW 6:21

Sweet Sam

Good afternoon, God!

My morning started with a bolt out of bed! I had a 9:00 a.m. meeting at the medical center with the hospice director regarding Mom's care, and I woke up at 8:00! Time for half a cup of coffee, quick shower, minimal makeup, and my go-to random clothing choices.

I talked to You on the way to the hospital. Sang to You as I looked at the beautiful art displayed in the heavens. Rain began to gently fall from the sky. I did mention I missed You and would like to "hear" from You. To feel loved and comforted in an earthly and tangible way.

My sister and Director Dave were chatting with Mom when I arrived. Choosing our words carefully, cheerfully, and cautiously, we presented the benefits of hospice, and the steps we needed to take in preparation for the move home.

So much of the conversation was familiar, stored in my brain and heart. Stinging facts, choices, and decisions. Memories of Jack's adventures with hospice and caregiving, I never dreamed I'd be revisiting this world so soon. Medications, machines, schedules, doctors, nurses, aides, equipment. I sat discussing words and phrases of the recent past from another time, another place, another person I loved with my whole being. Similar sounds and plans. The known and unknown. Mom will be going home today, and when she heard the news, the cute smile I've seen my entire life appeared across her oxygen-tubed face.

After our meeting, we scurried our separate ways with assignments to accomplish for Mom's move.

I was famished, so I stopped at the local café for an egg over medium, a piece of whole-wheat toast, and a cup of black tea. I sat and stared, letting the morning conversations and decisions soak in, much like the soft rain. I kept reminding myself I was smack dab in the middle of a busy restaurant and crying was not allowed. I felt tears welling up inside, ready to escape at any moment. To prevent this spectacle, I bit my lower lip to divert my attention from tears to pain. It works for me.

After I ate, I gathered my handbag, umbrella, car keys, and ticket. I stood in line behind all the others waiting their turn to pay. My mind was a bit foggy, I gazed ahead, not noticing anyone in particular. A voice from behind me asked, "Do you have a job?" I turned to see an elderly man directly behind me. His small body was bent over and propped up with a sturdy wooden cane. He had suspenders attached to his trousers. A plaid shirt was tucked under a bright red fleece jacket. His eyes were blue, his smile was warm, and he was looking directly into my soul. I explained my job was taking care of my mother at the moment. He reached for my ticket to pay my bill, and when I objected, he said, "God told me to do this."

How could I argue with a proclamation from "on high?" I started to cry (of course). I walked to my table to leave a tip for the waitress and to gather my composure, then back to say thank you, again. I introduced myself, and he told me his name was Sam. I will always remember him as Sweet Sam.

Jesus in disguise was my first impression of this angelic man. I reached for his hand and was astonished at the strength and warmth of his handshake. Well, it was really more of a handhold. His grip was not what I expected at all, but then again, I felt his soulful power from the moment I turned to see Sam's crystal blue eyes and easy smile. He said, "Have a blessed day." He was my blessed day.

I cried all the way home, the type of tears I had repressed at the restaurant were replaced with new and improved happy tears.

As I drove, I remembered the setting and the people gathered in little tables and booths eating their brunch. I had dressed up for our hospital meeting. My bright Kelly-green shirt, black pants, patent leather sandals. Adorned myself with dangling gold earrings, a dainty gold and soft pastel necklace. Plus, three gold bracelets, and a pearl ring on my freshly manicured hand, gifts Jack had given to me over the years. I was decked out. Yes, they were my random clothes selection of the day, but they were from my go-to emergency cute stash.

I was reminded this was another part of the miracle. An onlooker would have believed I should be buying Sweet Sam *his* meal. No matter how we appear on the outside, You see the inner depths of our being. Yes, I could have paid for both of our meals that day. You had different plans for each of us. I wasn't starving for food, I was starving for Your touch, and You sent Sam to let me know You heard my prayer and nourished my soul.

You amaze me! Your timing is impeccable. Your gifts are perfect.

I honestly will love You . . . Forever and a Day!
Love, Debby

*He has put his angels in charge of you
to watch over you wherever you go.*
—PSALM 91:11

Missing My Man

Good morning, God!

I miss Jack!!

The past few years I've been busy, so utterly consumed with his care that I pretty much forgot our lives before Parkinson's and Lewy Body Dementia.

The last few days I've been blessed with wonderful memories of life with Jack, as a couple. Not as caregiver and patient, but an awesomely crazy-in-love couple. Kissing, holding hands, playing golf, dancing. Our wedding day, honeymoon, and anniversaries. Trips with friends. Family celebrations.

Thank You for letting those memories resurface. The images in my head have been so vivid and the love in my heart so real. I've also been sad. A deep, quiet, way past your heart kind of sadness.

Realizing that spending the rest of my life with the man I love is not a possibility, not a reality, not even a hope. It's not to be.

I miss Jack, I miss what we had, and I miss what will never be. My mind doesn't know how to rest. My body doesn't remember how to sleep. I thought after Jack came to be with You I would be able to breathe and quiet my thoughts.

Help me understand this new life of mine. Stay by my side.

Thank You for sending such sweet "couple memories" of my ruggedly handsome husband.

I love you both so much!
Forever and a Day,
Debby

Sometimes you will never know the value of a moment until it becomes a memory.

—Dr. Seuss

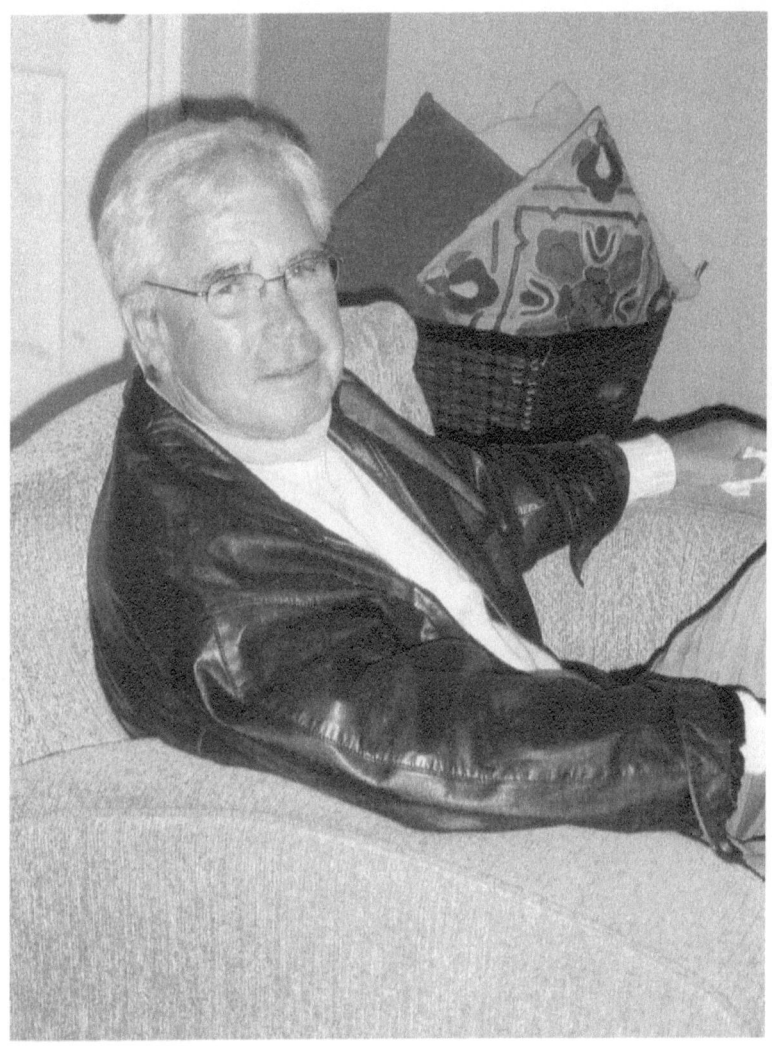

A Hole in My Heart

Good morning, God!

    A hole in my heart.
    That's the way my parents explained the defect I was born with. The reason my lips and fingers turned blue. The reason for myriad doctors' appointments. The need for needles and injections. Drinking and swallowing gross white chalky mixtures. The importance of strange machines and cold x-ray slides attached to my body. The reason for open heart surgery.
    I was six years old. My surgery to correct ventricular septal defect and pulmonary stenosis was scheduled for the following year. The year of 1960.
    I trusted my parents. They taught me to trust You. We attended attended church prayer service every Wednesday evening at 7:00. After the meeting, my mom and dad would take me to the preachers of our church. I would sit in a "big girl" chair. The ministers were dressed in nice suits and pretty ties. They would place their hands on my head and talk to You about me and about my surgery. My parents would stand close, bow their heads, and close their eyes.
    A warm, loving feeling would fill my damaged heart, and I would know without a doubt I was safe. I was happy. I was carefree. I was covered by a spirit of peace. At the age of six I didn't have the words to describe my thoughts, but now I do.
    A hole in my heart.
    Parents, prayers.

Doctors, nurses.
The Great Physician.
Perfect healing.
A whole heart!

Thank You for mending my heart over and over throughout the years. Scars cover my body. Some are visible, others only You and I know about. Places You have touched and patched. Scars remain, but I am healed once again. My heart has a steady, strong beat.

I *still* ache for Jack.

Heartache.

You continue to do Your magic. Your seamless inner stitching. Once again, my heart is on the mend. I'm in the care of my Creator.

Forever and a Day,
Debby

He heals up the broken-hearted and binds up their wounds.
—Psalm 147:3

The hands that made the stars are holding your heart.
—Psalm 139:13

A Little Weepy

Good morning, God!

    I'm a little weepy this morning.
    I continue to be stuck in the days of confusion.
    One minute I believe with all my heart I have my path figured out, then the bottom drops out of all my plans.
    I've seen and felt grief, pain, agony, doubt, and now I feel my mind and my heart are fixed in the deep currents of confusion. I've never been a good swimmer—not even mediocre. I can barely dogpaddle. I'm *drowning* in confusion. How do I free myself and rise above these waves? What do I do? Where do I *go?* Who am I? How do I find You?
    Guess I should cry out to the One Who Walks On Water. Hey, my mind and heart may be floating a bit after this realization. Funny how I forget Your power and promises, thus the flailing and sinking begins.
    Light-bulb moment! Even though I'm a terrible swimmer, I know and love and adore the One Who Walks On Water. I am reminded my eyes must be on You or the waters will be too deep and the storms too fierce and I *will* sink.
    Then I hear Your voice, and You reach out Your hand, pulling me to safety.
    Just remembering this helps the weeping subside, calmness return, confusion vanish.
    I still don't have all the answers to all my questions; however, I

know who does, and that knowledge definitely calms the waves and keeps me afloat.

This tiny conversation with You has made a monumental difference in my day.

Thanks for Your promises and Your presence.

All My Love—
Forever and a Day,
Debby

He reached down from heaven and rescued me;
he drew me out of deep waters.
—PSALM 18:16

Holidays

Good evening, God!

Holidays bring out emotions I didn't know I had. I am astounded with the sudden bursts of tears and laughter and bah-humbugs. One big fat conglomeration of ups and downs.

Last year I was trying with all my might to make November, December, and January festive, jolly, and bright. Jack, my sweet husband, passed away October 14. As I said, I tried and succeeded in many ways, with the help and happiness of family, friends, and strangers in celebrating the miracle of the season. This year I am again trying with all my might to make November, December, and January festive, jolly, and bright. My sweet Mom passed away October 28. Unexpected tears have been abundant. Smiles seem much easier than laughter and I guess I'll depend on family, friends, and strangers to help me again this year. I know there is magic this time of year, and I long to see it. I want to be part of the real world and the future, while remembering the beauty of the past.

I *love* illuminating lights during the holidays. Lifting my spirits with twinkling white lights . . . I love that idea! The white lights are the present I'll give to myself. Strands of glowing bulbs to hang from the wooden beams on my cozy patio. Reminding me when the skies are dark I can hang a few glass bobbles, plug in wishes, and breathe in joy. This is definitely a good start.

May I remember You and Your majesty, love, forgiveness, and encouragement. May I feel Your warm and brilliant light wrapped around me during the season of new birth, new hope, and new dreams.

Thank You for Jesus.
Thank You for Jack.
Thank You for Mom.
Holidays in heaven . . . hallelujah.

Happy holidays to all.
And to all a very good night.
Forever and a Day,
Debby

I pray that the God who gives hope
will fill you with much joy and peace while you trust in him!
Then your hope will overflow by the power of the Holy Spirit.
—ROMANS 12:12

Crazy?!

Good morning, God!

Crazies in grief!

I'm beginning to worry about my sanity. I know this concern should have set in a few years back. I described myself back then as fun and quirky. To reiterate, concern has set in!

A few examples include... putting both contacts in the same eye and wondering why the world is lopsided.

Applying *all* my makeup and *then* getting in the shower. Not knowing what I had done, until I freaked out from the black streaks running down my chest, suddenly recognizing the color of mascara "midnight noir." Only then did I awaken to my insanity.

Walking out the door in frigid weather and wondering why there was such a chill. Accessing the situation . . . Shirt, yes. Underwear, yes. Opaque black tights with socks, yes. Sweater-coat, yes. Boots, yes. Missing? My black skinny pants!

There are hundreds of examples of the crazy things I am still doing one year and two months after Jack has moved on to his mansion in the sky. These things, until now, have only been shared with my sister and my two daughters and occasionally my two best friends (thank goodness, I only have two). It's a miracle someone hasn't come to my front door to escort me to a place of safety for myself and for others.

This Christmas my sister's gift to me included four sessions with a shrink. I'm not kidding. It is funny and sad at the same time and pretty pitiful. Oh well, four sessions wrapped up in a big beautiful red satin bow! Merry Christmas to me.

Now, back to reasons for my entry into the witness protection program.

Experts in the field of grief tell me, "You're not going crazy, it's just part of the process." Okay, I feel better. Then the experts continue (when they should just stop and move on to another uplifting fact) and tell me the psycho lady living inside me could stay for years. Now, isn't that special?

Thank You for the extraordinary people you have placed in my life to help me along the way to health and happiness . . . sisters, daughters, family, friends, and yes, even shrinks. They truly make my life sweeter.

Forever and a Day,
Debby

I live in my own little world, but it's ok.
They know me here!
—Lauren Myracle

One Regret

Good morning, God.

I wake up early each morning and open my eyes to the ceiling staring back at me. Stretch my legs and raise my arms toward the "sky." My brain begins to unwind with the beat of the twirling fan directly over my head.

I lie in bed and remember that I'm alone. No one is lying next to me. Next to me lie five neatly lined pillows on Jack's side of the bed, which is my attempt to find comfort. I close my eyes again. This morning my mind is reliving the biggest regret in loving Jack. My biggest regret is not letting Jack "go" on his own terms.

I tried desperately to take care of him and to wait for the "coming soon" cure. There were well-known, wealthy people working diligently to find the miracle meds or treatment that would finally heal my husband and I convinced myself we just needed to hang on a little bit longer. Michael J. Fox, Muhammad Ali, Billy Graham. Help was on the way.

I researched, read, studied, attended classes and seminars. Anticipating the cure. I made appointments with expert physicians in the field of neurology. I discussed, argued, questioned, suggested, pleaded with nurses and doctors for answers and hope. Jack's primary physician was in Houston. So, we fought the I-10 traffic, dodging never-ending eighteen-wheelers and non-stop construction. Our two-and-a-half-hour drive to the specialist was always eventful and memorable.

He also had local docs and appointments scheduled on a regular and as-needed basis.

Hospital stays, rehab facilities, long-term care outings, and nursing home visits. These times became more frequent as the years and disease progressed. But, he always came home at some point. Home to me. And we were "us" once again.

Year seven was a turning point. His hallucinations and delusions were 24/7 and out of control. Paranoia, violence, and hysteria were "normal" and unrelenting. His blood pressure fluctuated dramatically. He was admitted to a local hospital that Father's Day and stayed for two months. He moved from a regular room to the long-term care unit and finally to Ten Tower. Regret took my breath away and my sleep, but not my tears—they were a constant.

As a result of the two-month stay, his Houston physician came up with a medicine regime that worked . . . to a degree. Our options had been depleted, so we followed the doctor's treatment plan, packed our bags, and found our way home.

Jack had blood drawn each and every week because of the serious side effects of his new magic med: clozapine. Lab results faxed from the Louisiana lab to the Houston doctor and then back to the Louisiana pharmacy. All for seven pills, and the "joy" of "same time next week." You heard my constant weekly prayers that each facet of the process would be seamless and completed in a timely fashion. Seven pills were essential for halfway "happy hallucinations" and "diminished delusions."

Why didn't I let him die on his own terms? He told me about year four he wanted to die one of two ways. He said, "I'd like to go either of a heart attack or heat exhaustion on the golf course with my buddies after eighteen bogey-free holes or overdosing on Viagra—but preferably Cialis—with you by my side!" No joking. No sarcasm. Just truth.

Why didn't I allow him to die on his own terms? Why did I try so desperately to keep him alive to wait for the cure?

I couldn't have helped with the golf course request, except I guess, technically, I could have dropped him off at the club one summer day and allowed the Louisiana humidity and heat to do their work. Jack would have been happy, excited, and content.

I didn't need to confiscate his little blue or yellow pills. At the time, I thought I did. His disease kept his blood pressure in a constant state of upheaval. When he took his favorite pills, his pressure would plummet, he would pass out, and then become ill for several days. Many times, I honestly believed he *had* died, and his dreams had come to fruition. He proved me wrong time and time again. Resurrection was his. So, I hid them to protect him and to save him. For what? From what? Years of illness, suffering, pain?

These thoughts twirl around and around in my mind, like the ceiling fan over my head. Make them *stop!* I crawl out of bed to redirect my thoughts, change the scenery, and search for You.

Other regrets come to mind, but this one haunts me still.

If I had do-overs, the key to his golf cart would *always* have been in the ignition and ready for takeoff. Blue and yellow pills would have been placed on his bedside table in plain view without the child-safety cap intact. *His* choices to make.

His own terms. His own way. His own time.

Did I love him too tightly—too intensely?

Maybe so. Probably so.

My greatest regret.

I'm so sorry Jack.

Please forgive me.

Forever and a Day,
I love You Lord,
I love you, Jack.
Debby

*Did all your experience mean nothing at all?
Surely it meant something!*
—Galatians 3:4

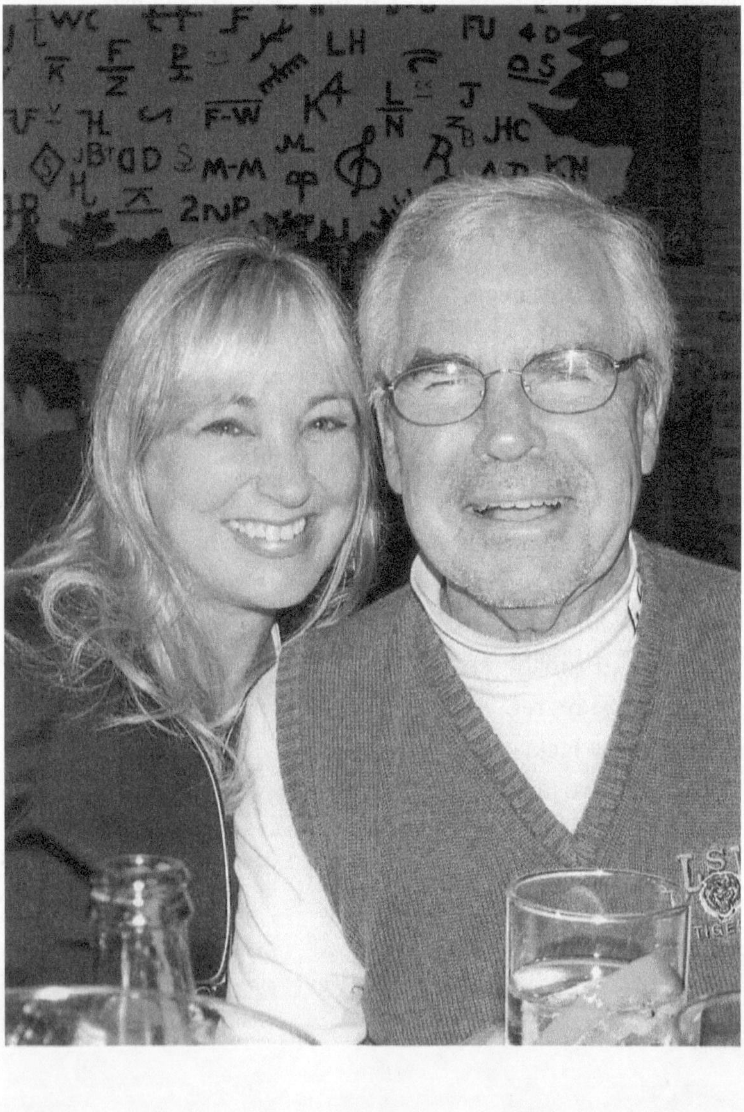

Sacred, Specific Scriptures

Good evening, God!

This morning as I was flipping through my journal, I stumbled across a letter I had written to You five years ago. At the time, I thought I had nothing to offer—just empty hands. I felt my path was blocked by disease, illness, and limitations. You gave me the gift of this verse . . . Matthew 25:35–36.

"I was hungry, and you gave me food. I was thirsty, and you gave me something to drink. I was alone, and away from home, and you invited me into your home. I was without clothes, and you gave me something to wear. *I was sick, and you cared for me.* I was in prison, and you visited me."

The phrase You stated, "I was sick, and you cared for me," was a wow moment for me. You saw my reaction! I could have done cartwheels right then and there. Maybe a handstand! You get the idea. I took that verse and ran with it—a purpose, a plan, and a passion. I began to care for my husband in an entirely different light. In caring for him, I was caring for You and serving You. Two for the price of one. Double delight!

Over the years I would recite this golden nugget whenever the road was becoming hard to travel. Reminding myself I was making a difference. My hands were busy serving my two favorite fellows.

As I was rereading verses 35–36 this morning, my eyes and

spirit were opened more completely. I was astonished, amazed, and grateful.

Cartwheels. Handstands. Hallelujahs!

You allowed me to see the complete picture. The fact that in helping and caring for my husband over the span of fourteen years, I fulfilled each and every act of love in these preciously precise verses for my wonderfully wonderful Jack.

He was *hungry*, and I prepared and fed him his favorite foods. Plenty of ice cream!

He was *thirsty*, and I helped him drink green tea from his LSU cup.

He was a *stranger* and couldn't find his way "home." I took him in and tucked him in.

He was *naked*, and I dressed him for the day and pjs for the night. Extra blankets!

He was *sick*, and I loved, kissed, hugged, and cared for him.

He was in his own painful *prison*. I stayed with him day and night.

I've come a *long* way since "I was sick, and you cared for me." Thank You for showing me how to give "all of me."

I honestly don't have the words to express my love for You, my best friend but You already know. I like that about You.

Night. Sweet dreams.

Forever and a Day,
And another day . . .
Debby

Is That Me?

Good morning, God!

I looked in the mirror this morning and was pleasantly surprised! The person staring back at me was familiar and her name was on the tip of my tongue.

Perhaps an acquaintance, or an old friend from long ago.

I walked in the bedroom and picked up a gold-framed image of one I had known from the past and carried it to the mirror. I placed the "framed friend" next to me. Side by side, we both stared at our reflections. She smiled. She was *always* smiling, tucked in her golden frame. I began to cry. Happy tears, thankful tears, amazed tears. We both began to grin from ear to ear. A similar look! An identical smile!

The person in the mirror had a slight twinkle in her eyes. Definite smile on her lips. Shine in her "just slept on" messy blonde hair. A few well-earned wrinkles on her rosy soft skin. Who was this gorgeous "girl" in the mirror? She was a vision! God woke up early and encircled a heavenly glow around my friend from the past. She was radiant.

I recognized her once again, after all these years . . . Debby. It's really her! It's unmistakably me! Not my "old" self, but my "new-old" self. Vastly improved.

Thank You for rest and healing.

Thank You for introducing me to my new and improved self. Thank You, I'm "lookin' good!" Well . . . better. I'll take it.

Almost two years have passed. I never imagined I would encounter this "cutie pie" again. For years I consciously avoided reflections of her, now I catch myself gazing in disbelief at the pretty lady in the mirror smiling back at me. What a blessing! What a miracle!

Thank You for reminding me I am beautiful in Your sight. Thank You for loving me back to health and happiness.

Loving You . . .
Forever and a Day!
"Cutie Pie"

*Just when the Caterpillar
Thought the world was over,
It became a Butterfly.*
—PROVERB

Happiness is the best facelift.
—DIANA KRALL

The Beginning, Again

Good morning, God!

It's a beautiful, cool October day. The temperature is in the low seventies. The sun is golden, warm, and in full-shine mode. Don't You just love it when *I* give *You* the weather report!

Finished a brisk walk at our neighborhood park. Yes, You heard correctly. I've walked two days in a row. Yes, a minor miracle. Haven't worked up a sweat yet, don't want to freak my body out the first week of exercise. Easing my way back to a healthy body and fitted pants.

Your park was spectacular! Where did You come up with such a plethora of colors? Trees covered in tangerine orange, pineapple yellow, and candy red. Showing off their fancy new hairdos. Emerald green grass fresh with the sparkle of morning dew. Baby blue skies, with streaks of white clouds. Rays in soft pinks and deep lavenders bridging heaven and earth. Flowers too intricate to describe adequately. I just sigh, sing, and soak it in.

October is one of my favorite times of year. The trail at the park exploded with vibrant vivid colors. Around every corner magical hues emerged. You must be so proud. I bet this is one of Your favorite seasons, too.

As I walked, I talked to You about this particular month, this time of year, and my memories.

October is an exceptional month.

October is the month Jack and I spotted each other for the first time, years ago.

October is the month we continue to celebrate Jack's birthday. October 22.

October is the month he spent his first heavenly birthday with You. October 14.

October is a perfect month for new beginnings.

My spirit is happy, energized, and invigorated as I remember the park-path stroll.

My memories are light, beautiful, and magnificent.

Just like Your creation.

Just like October. Just like Jack.

Just like You!

Walking the path made me aware of Your presence. And not today alone. Your presence during our entire journey in "sickness and in health." Through the years of commitment to each other, come rain or shine. You were an ever-present source of comfort and strength, winter, spring, summer, and fall. I'm not going to try to make a list of all You were to us, but simply and completely expressed *You were our everything.*

I'm sure Jack has already thanked You because he is still a Southern Gentleman. I wonder how he expressed his thanks? Jitterbug is his specialty. On second thought, I imagine him standing before You and speaking his praise and appreciation. As You know, Jack had struggled to speak since birth and the disease took even that away from him. Now, for the first time in his life he can talk without a speech impediment... no stuttering involved! That makes me smile. Visualizing that moment makes me "sadappy." A word I contrived to convey my duo feelings of sad and happy at the exact same time. Yep, I'm still creative and crazy.

I will thank You the rest of this earthly life. I'm saving a *huge* hug for You when I finish the journey. When I cross the threshold. So, be prepared!

Cheers to You!

I'm stronger because of You.

I'm excited because of You.
I'm humbled because of You.
Thank You, God!

Please take my hand as I begin again. I'm ready. As long as I feel the warmth of Your hand holding mine. A new adventure. A new beginning. Please walk with me. I'm still a little nervous.

I have Your number.
I know Your name.
I'll talk to You tomorrow.

> Forever and forever and forever . . . and a day
> My love for You!
> Debby

O Lord, Our Lord
how majestic is your name in all the earth!
—Psalm 8:9

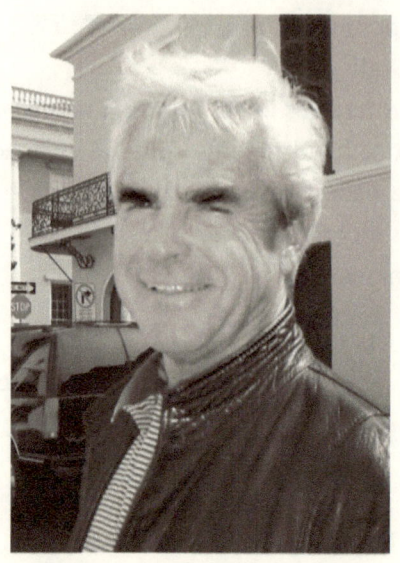

You changed my sorrow into dancing.
You took away my clothes of sadness,
and clothed me in happiness.
I will sing to you and not be silent.
Lord, my God, I will praise you forever (and a day).
—Psalm 30:11–12

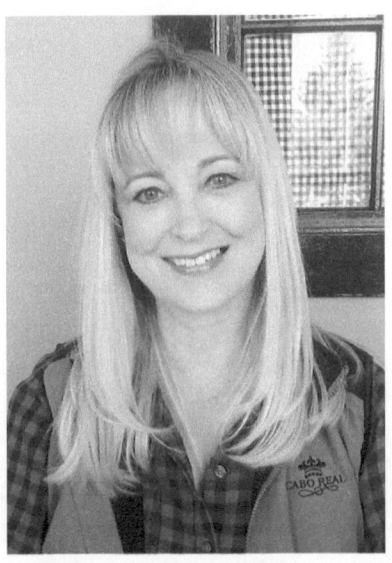

DEBBY JONES WORLEY was born in the heart of Oklahoma, grew up surrounded by the tumbleweeds of west Texas, and found her way to the swamplands of Louisiana. In Louisiana she fell in love with Cajun cuisine, soulful jazz, LSU purple and gold, and the wonderfully unique people. She calls Lake Charles home.

She is blessed with beautiful children, grandchildren, family, and friends from the mountains of Montana across the plains of Texas to the bayous of Louisiana.

She speaks from her heart. She relies on words and whispers from her Heavenly Father. She prays her letters will offer comfort, joy, and hope.

WOULD YOU BE SO KIND as to leave a book review? Authors' books have a much better chance at being successful when the readers share that they've enjoyed reading the book . . . which I hope you did. Doing so will mean that far more people will potentially see the book and, I hope, be lifted up in their relationship with God.

If you could take those few minutes to leave a review, I'd appreciate it ever so much.

www.ingramcontent.com/pod-product-compliance
Lightning Source LLC
Chambersburg PA
CBHW020122130526
44591CB00032B/382